How to Conduct Behavioral Research over the Internet

Methodology in the Social Sciences

David A. Kenny, *Series Editor*

PRINCIPLES AND PRACTICE OF STRUCTURAL EQUATION MODELING
  Rex B. Kline

SPECTRAL ANALYSIS OF TIME-SERIES DATA
  Rebecca M. Warner

A PRIMER ON REGRESSION ARTIFACTS
  Donald T. Campbell and David A. Kenny

REGRESSION ANALYSIS FOR CATEGORICAL MODERATORS
  Herman Aguinis

HOW TO CONDUCT BEHAVIORAL RESEARCH OVER THE INTERNET
A BEGINNER'S GUIDE TO HTML AND CGI/PERL
  R. Chris Fraley

How to Conduct Behavioral Research over the Internet

A Beginner's Guide to HTML and CGI/Perl

R. Chris Fraley

SERIES EDITOR'S NOTE by David A. Kenny

gp

THE GUILFORD PRESS
New York   London

© 2004 The Guilford Press
A Division of Guilford Publications, Inc.
72 Spring Street, New York, NY 10012
www.guilford.com

Printed in the United States of America

This book is printed on acid-free paper.

Last digit is print number: 9 8 7 6 5 4 3 2 1

Library of Congress Cataloging-in-Publication Data

Fraley, R. Chris.
  How to conduct behavioral research over the internet : a beginner's
    guide to HTML and CGI/PERL / R. Chris Fraley.
      p. cm. — (Methodology in the social sciences)
    Includes bibliographical references and index.
    1-57230-997-0 (pbk.)
    1. Internet research. 2. Psychology—Research—Methodology.
  3. Social sciences—Research—Methodology. 4. Psychology—Research—
  Data processing. 5. Social sciences—Research—Data processing.
  6. HTML (Document markup language) 7. CGI (Computer network
  protocol)   8. Perl (Computer program language)   I. Title.
  II. Series.
  BF76.6.I57F73 2004
  150′.285′4678—dc22

                                                    2003027516

About the Author

R. Chris Fraley received his PhD in social–personality psychology from the University of California, Davis. He conducts research on attachment theory and close relationships, personality development, and emotion regulation. He is currently Assistant Professor of Psychology at the University of Illinois.

Series Editor's Note

How to Conduct Behavioral Research over the Internet, by R. Chris Fraley, is a welcome addition to the Methodology in the Social Sciences series. This is the first book in the series that has focused on a particular way to gather data rather than on the statistical analysis of data after they are gathered; it is certainly as important a topic. For many readers, *How to Conduct Behavioral Research over the Internet* will provide a new way to collect data.

The way social scientists have viewed the Internet has changed over the years. Those of us who have been working for 20 or more years remember the early Internet as a mail service. It put us in immediate contact with colleagues all over the world. However, before the advent of browsers and web pages, the early Internet was more of a curiosity than a research tool. Eventually, though, it did become a source of information—both useful and useless—on research topics. Most of us don't think past that as a role for the Internet in research. As this book describes, however, the Internet has another purpose, and one that might eventually become even more important for researchers than information gathering (especially given how much misinformation there is on the Web): the Internet as a source of data.

I had my own epiphany regarding the usefulness of the Internet for data collection when I saw the marvelous study conducted by Robins, Trzesniewski, Tracy, Gosling, and Potter (2002) on developmental changes in self-esteem. Only by using the Internet did these researchers obtain a sample from all over the world with 326,000 participants, ages 9 to 90! They were able to document the changes in self-esteem as a function of age, gender, and ethnicity. Significance tests weren't particularly necessary when dealing with over a quarter million participants.

But how would *we* conduct a research study like that of Robins et al.? R. Chris Fraley has written a book that shows how. This book and the website he has developed in conjunction with it (www.web-research-design. net—from which it is intended that readers will download the code presented herein) provide the means for conducting this type of research. An impressive feature is that the book is comprehensible to those who have never created a web page and to those who do not consider themselves programmers (almost all of us). Moreover, the book does not just show how to conduct surveys on the Internet, it provides details on how to conduct experiments. It shows how to randomize the presentation of stimuli, measure reaction times, provide immediate feedback, and so on. Finally, the book has many useful hints for how to make data analysis easier and simpler. One wonders if we are not too far away from having a program that will write our results section for us.

Even those who do not plan to conduct this type of research will benefit from reading this book. First, we are all consumers of research and to be knowledgeable consumers, it is helpful to see how such research is conducted. The book certainly provides such a picture. Second, if we wanted to use the Internet for teaching, rather than for research, for instance, much of what the book details would be of great usefulness in teaching and evaluating students. That is, the techniques here would be easily modifiable for any number of purposes.

I think *How to Conduct Behavioral Research over the Internet* is a path-setting book. It will give many of us a boost into data collection in the 21st century.

Reference

Robins, R. W., Trzesniewski, K. H., Tracy, J. L., Gosling, S. D., & Potter, J. (2002). Global self-esteem across the lifespan. *Psychology and Aging, 17,* 423–434.

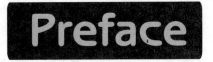

Preface

My personal interest in Internet research began in the late 1990s. As a social–personality psychologist, a substantial portion of my research is focused on assessing individual differences among people, and trying to understand the mechanisms and processes underlying those differences. In my research on adult attachment patterns (see Fraley & Shaver, 2000), my colleagues and I have used self-report questionnaires to assess variability in how secure or insecure people feel in their close relationships. However, the inevitable process of administering questionnaires, entering the data by hand into Microsoft Excel or SPSS (Statistical Package for Social Science), and managing all the paperwork proved to be time-consuming. It made sense to find a way to automate the process as much as possible. Moreover, to make it more satisfying for my research subjects, I wanted them to be able to get instantaneous feedback on how they scored on the questionnaires.

Although I knew it was possible to accomplish these goals by using the Internet, I didn't know how to pull it off. I spent a considerable amount of time browsing the computer sections of bookstores in hope of finding something like *Internet Research for Dummies*. No such book exists. I was eventually able to figure out how to make online surveys by studying (i.e., dissecting and tweaking) existing web pages that contained questionnaire items. I also learned a lot from reading online tutorials about "HTML Forms" (which we'll discuss in Chapter 4). But I still didn't know how to store the data collected from these questionnaires, or how to get the web page to score someone's responses and explain to the participant what those responses might mean. By dissecting still more pages, I eventually learned that standard web pages can't perform these tasks and that I would need to work with dynamic programs called *CGI scripts* that run on a *server* in order to accomplish my goals.

Any introductions I did find to the topic of online psychological research were overly broad, surveying many of the possible tools that could be used, but leaving the reader unable to actually *do* anything particularly useful. On the other hand, books that explain CGI programming in depth are not written with the researcher in mind.

My objective in writing this book was to create a basic, step-by-step guide for social scientists who are interested in using the Internet to conduct research. This book has been written to be a one-stop shop, if you will, for creating innovative and functional studies online from the ground up. Any researcher with access to nothing more than a desktop computer, a healthy dose of curiosity and patience—and this book—should be able to conduct online research within a couple of weeks.

In this book I begin by showing you how to set up a web server and design rudimentary web pages in HTML. Next, I introduce CGI programming in Perl—the real guts of the book. CGI programs are designed to run on a web server, and, unlike standard HTML web pages, these programs can be used to create a dynamic, interactive web experience for the user. By using CGI programs, researchers can randomize the presentation order of stimuli, randomly assign subjects to conditions, automatically save response data to files for data analysis, provide subjects with customized feedback based on their responses, utilize both text and image-based stimuli, measure response times, and employ complex branching operations within a project. These are the subjects covered in Chapters 5 through 14. Each chapter presents one or two examples of how to implement a "generic" research technique (i.e., random assignment), explains the code in depth, and describes how the code can be tailored to different applications. The final chapter of the book reviews some of the advantages and disadvantages of web research.

This book is intended for anyone who currently conducts or is interested in conducting research in the social and behavioral sciences (e.g., psychology, sociology, epidemiology, economics, anthropology, marketing). Although many of the techniques and applications I discuss focus on psychological applications, nonpsychologists should have no trouble understanding how these tools would be modified to serve their purposes.

I would like to express my gratitude to Michael Birnbaum, John Krantz, Gary McClelland, Ken McGraw, Ulf Reips, and William Schmidt for organizing the National Science Foundation-sponsored *Advanced Training Institute for Social Psychology Experiments via the WWW*, held in January 2002. I learned an extraordinary amount from this crew, and I'd like to thank them for taking the time to organize the workshop and sharing their knowledge. I would especially like to thank Billy Schmidt for showing me how to set up a web server and teaching me the basics of Perl. If it weren't for Billy, I would have been wandering from one dead end to another for a long time. I would also like to thank my students and colleagues for encouraging me to write this book. I have written it with them in mind, and I hope they will not only learn a lot from it, but enjoy reading it as well. I thank David Mitchell at The Guilford Press for his extensive work with the book. I'm grateful that he was brave enough to learn Perl in the process of editing the book; his feedback has made the book much clearer than it was in its first draft. Finally, I'd like to thank my wife, Caroline Tancredy, for patiently reading drafts of this book and pushing me to explain as clearly as possible the logic of the CGI programming.

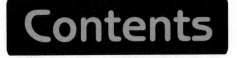

Contents

CHAPTER 1   **Introduction**   1

What You Will Be Able to Accomplish / 3
What You Will Need / 4
Some (Very) Basic Things You Need to Know
  about the Internet / 4
How to Get the Most Out of This Book / 6

CHAPTER 2   **Getting Started: A Step-by-Step Guide**   9
              to Using a Web Server

Method 1: Using a Professional Web Hosting Service / 11
  Signing Up with Netfirms / 12
  Transferring Files to Your Netfirms Server / 13
  Downloading and Installing WS_FTP Pro / 13
  Configuring WS_FTP Pro / 14
  Using WS_FTP Pro to Transfer Files / 15
  Creating a Data Directory / 18
  Some Important Notes on the Organization and Operation
    of Your Server / 19
      The Location of Your Web Pages / 19
      The Address or URL for Your Web Page / 19
      The CGI Folder / 20

Transferring Files / 20
Timing Out / 20
Method 2: Setting Up Your Own Server / 21
*Downloading and Installing Microsoft's Windows
Installer / 22*
Downloading and Installing ActivePerl / 23
Downloading and Installing the Apache Server / 24
Getting Your Server Up and Running / 26
Creating a Data Directory / 27
*Some Important Notes about the Organization and Operation
of Your Server / 28*
Transferring Files to the Server / 28
The Location of Your Web Pages / 29
The Address or URL for Your Web Pages / 29
The CGI Folder / 30
Turning On and Turning Off the Server / 30
Troubleshooting / 31

CHAPTER 3   HTML: How to Make a Web Page from Scratch   33

Downloading and Installing 1st Page / 35
What Is Required in All HTML Pages / 36
Creating Text / 37
Page Properties / 38
Formatting Text / 41
Bold / 41
Italics / 41
Font / 41
Text Size / 42
Text Color / 42
Line Spacing / 42
Centering Text / 43
Blank Space / 43
Inserting an Image / 44
Creating Hyperlinks / 48
Using Images as Links / 49
Using Tables Effectively / 50
Bringing It All Together / 53
Summary / 56

CHAPTER 4   **HTML Forms: Collecting Research Data**   60
from Participants via the Internet

The Form Tag / 61
Creating Response Windows and Rating Scales / 62
   Text Boxes / 62
   Radio Buttons / 64
   Pull-Down Menus / 66
   Checkboxes / 68
The **Submit** Button / 69
Image Maps / 69
Hidden Tags / 70
Two Examples / 71

CHAPTER 5   **An Introduction to CGI Scripting: Using Perl**   82
to Automatically Save Response Data to a File

Saving the Data via a Simple CGI Script / 86
   The First Line of All Perl Scripts / 87
   Instructing the Server to Process the Submitted Data / 87
   Extracting Values from the Submitted Data and Assigning Them
      Variable Names within the CGI Script / 88
   Writing to a Data File / 89
   Inserting HTML Code into the CGI Script / 91
Testing the Code / 92
Example 2: Time Stamping a Submission / 95
   Time Stamp / 96
   Environmental Variables / 97
Let's See It Work / 98
Importing the Data into SPSS / 98
Summary / 99

CHAPTER 6   **Providing Customized Feedback**   104
to Research Participants

Providing Feedback: Averaging a User's Responses / 105
Providing Feedback: Averaging a User's Responses and Saving
   the Data / 110
Data Analysis on the Server: Averaging the Responses
   of Everyone in Your Sample / 112

Using If–Else Conditionals to Tailor the Feedback
 Further / 117
Sample Size and Feedback / 121
Summary / 123

CHAPTER 7   **Randomizing the Order of Stimuli**   **126**

An Illustration / 127
For–Next Loops / 129
Breaking Down the Code / 133
Processing and Saving Randomized Data / 136
Another Example, with a Slight Twist / 138
A Final Example, with a Bigger Twist / 142
Summary / 144

CHAPTER 8   **Random Assignment to Conditions**   **146**

An Example / 146
Another Way to Implement Random Assignment / 151
Manipulating Variables within-Subjects / 153
Summary / 153

CHAPTER 9   **Using Multiple Web Pages in Research:**   **155**
             Carrying Responses Forward from One Page
             to the Next

An Example / 156
Randomizing Trials across Multiple Web Pages / 162
Using Image Maps to Advance from One Page
 to the Next / 167
Summary / 173

CHAPTER 10   **Using Conditional Branching Structures:**   **174**
             An Example of "Skip Patterns"
             in Survey Research

Summary / 180

CHAPTER 11   **Advanced Feedback: Summarizing Data with Bar**   181
             Graphs and Two-Dimensional Plots

Bar Graphs / 182
Two-Dimensional Coordinate Graphs / 188
Summary / 198

CHAPTER 12   **Tracking Participants over Multiple Sessions:**   199
             PINs, Passwords, and Menus

An Example / 200
Dissecting the Code / 201
Customizing the Code / 213
Summary / 213

CHAPTER 13   **Measuring Response Times**   215

An Example: The Recall of Emotional Memories / 217
A More Complex Extension: Saving the Data and Analyzing It
    for the Participant / 224
Building on the Example: Randomizing Trial Orders / 226
Summary / 232

CHAPTER 14   **Additional Applications of Perl: Discussion Forums**   233
             and Scored Tests

Online Discussion Forum / 234
    The CGI Scripts and How They Work / 240
    Summary of the Online Forum Programs / 257
Online Quizzes / 258

CHAPTER 15   **Wrapping It Up**   268

Troubleshooting / 268
Getting Your Site Known / 272
Ethics / 274
Apache Server Maintenance / 275
Security: Protecting Your Server / 276
Security: Protecting Your Data / 278

Sampling Issues / 281
Dropout / 283
Data Quality Control / 284
Web Design / 285
  Screen Size / 285
  Figure–Ground Contrast / 286
  Don't Use JavaScript / 286
  Test Your Page in Different Browsers / 287
  Minimize the Need to Click and Scroll / 287
  Avoid Jargon / 287
  Avoid Using Plug-Ins / 288
  Make Your Site Look Professional / 288
Summary / 289

References   291

Index   293

To download the code presented in this book, and to look for updates on various procedures described herein, please visit the website the author has developed in conjunction with this book: www.web-research-design.net.

Chapter 1

Introduction

In the last few years, an increasing number of behavioral scientists have begun to use the World Wide Web as a tool for conducting psychological research. It is easy to understand the appeal of using the Web for research purposes. Just about any study that can be conducted via traditional pencil-and-paper methods can be implemented online, but without the hassles of explicit transcription or data entry, the scheduling of research participants, and paper costs. Moreover, researchers who use computers in their experiments for manipulating visual or narrative stimuli, randomizing trials, or creating customized assessments can easily implement their studies online. Finally, although researchers might use the Web to collect data from the same pool of undergraduates as they would if they weren't using the Web, there is the possibility of opening our laboratory doors to participants from all over the world.

Unfortunately, there are very few resources available to the behavioral scientist who wishes to create online research studies. One of the best books on the market, *Introduction to Behavioral Research on the Internet* by Michael Birnbaum, does an outstanding job at broadly reviewing many of the tools one might use for Internet research, but it only briefly mentions CGI (common gateway interface) programming—a technique that is useful for designing dynamic and interactive online research applications. Other texts, such as

CGI Programming 101 by Jacqueline Hamilton or *Perl and CGI for the World Wide Web* by Elizabeth Castro, are wonderful introductions to CGI programming but are not written with the research scientist in mind.

My objective in writing this book was to create a basic, step-by-step guide for behavioral researchers who are interested in using the Internet to conduct research. This book has been written to be a one-stop shop, if you will, for moving from "square one" to the point where you can create innovative and dynamic studies online. A researcher with access to nothing more than a desktop computer, an Internet connection, a healthy dose of curiosity and patience, and this book (of course) should be able to conduct online research within two weeks or less.

I thought it would be advantageous for researchers to have a thorough discussion of *one* way to do Internet research, a way that was simple, required as little a monetary investment as possible, wouldn't assume extensive or perhaps any programming knowledge, and wouldn't require asking favors from one's local computer guru. Therefore, in this book I focus on *server-side CGI programming in Perl*. (What this means will be explained in more depth below.) It is not my intent to review all the possible tools one could use to conduct online research (e.g., Java, JavaScript, ASP, PHP, C++). I have chosen a way that works for me, and have presented it here as simply as possible so that other researchers might take advantage of it. As a consequence, some of the programming code we discuss will not be the most beautiful or efficient code in the world. (If you don't know what it means to describe code as "beautiful," that is a good thing—you have not been corrupted yet.) The code we discuss, however, will be explained thoroughly and it will get the job done.

The intended audience for this book is anyone who currently conducts or is interested in conducting research in the social and behavioral sciences (e.g., psychology, sociology, epidemiology, economics, anthropology, marketing). As a psychologist, I have found it easiest to write this book as if I were writing it for my colleagues and students in psychology. However, many of the techniques and applications I discuss are not limited to psychology, and researchers from other disciplines should have no trouble understanding how these tools can be used to serve their purposes.

WHAT YOU WILL BE ABLE TO ACCOMPLISH

It is my intention to provide you with the skills and knowledge you need to design a wide array of online research studies. To accomplish this, examples have been selected that illustrate what I consider to be the *generic components* of research projects—techniques that are common to a wide variety of research designs and areas of investigation. Here is a brief sampling of some of the generic skills that you will learn from this book:

- You will learn how to create web-based questionnaires involving rating scales, free responses, pull-down menus, and checklists.
- You will learn how to write programs that will store participants' data automatically in a text file—a file that can be imported easily into commonly used statistical software packages and spreadsheets, such as Microsoft Excel, S-Plus, SAS (Statistical Application Software), or SPSS (Statistical Package for Social Science).
- You will learn how to provide response-specific stimuli or specially tailored stimuli for your participants. Moreover, you will learn how to write programs that process a participant's data and provide him or her with immediate feedback (e.g., whether he or she was correct, how he or she scored on a personality inventory).
- You will learn how to randomize the order of stimuli, whether those stimuli are images, text, or questionnaire items.
- You will learn how to randomly assign participants to conditions of an online experiment.
- You will learn how to carry a participant's responses forward from one web page to the next in studies that use multiple web pages.
- You will learn how to create online quizzes for students that are graded or scored by the web server. Also, I will show you how to create an online discussion forum with which you and your students or colleagues can exchange ideas.
- You will learn how to implement some basic graphing and data analytic techniques online.
- You will learn how to implement logins, personal identification numbers (PINs), and passwords so that the same participants can be studied over multiple sessions.
- You will learn how to assess response times online.

WHAT YOU WILL NEED

The only "thing" you will need to get up-and-running is a simple desktop computer in your lab, office, or home. I will assume that your computer is connected to the Internet, and that you can easily use it to surf the Web or check e-mail. I will also assume that your computer is running Microsoft Windows (95, 98, 2000, Me, XP) as its operating system. This, of course, is not a prerequisite for conducting research over the Web, but this book would be more difficult to read if I were trying to explain how to do things for both PC users and Macintosh users. (If you're an experienced Mac user, you should have no trouble adapting the instructions discussed in this book to a Macintosh environment.) You will also need some special software that can be downloaded for free online, and I'll show you how to do so in the next two chapters. It should go without saying that you should already have some experience using the Internet. If you use the Web to order books, check e-mail, or search for interesting articles, you'll be fine. I will also assume that you have a research background that includes at least an undergraduate course in research methods and statistics.

SOME (VERY) BASIC THINGS YOU NEED TO KNOW ABOUT THE INTERNET

There are some recurring terms and concepts you'll need to know in order to get the most out of this book. A *browser* is a program used to view web pages. The two most commonly used browsers are Netscape's Navigator and Microsoft's Internet Explorer. When you view a web page, several complex things take place beneath the surface that make this possible. First, when you type in a *URL* (universal resource locator) or web address (e.g., http://www.web-research-design.net/index.htm), your computer sends a request to another computer "located" at that address. This computer is often called a *server*, and its job is to receive such requests, and then "serve" the requested information back to you—the *user*.

More often than not, the kind of information that is sent to your browser is in the form of *hypertext markup language* or *HTML*. HTML has become a standard way of sharing information over the Internet. Your browser translates the HTML code that it receives from a server into the kinds of web pages with which we are familiar. The *World Wide Web* (WWW), by the way, is nothing more than the network of computers all over the world that participate in this process.

In your typical day-to-day experience with the Web, you probably do little more than view your favorite web pages or link from one page to another in hopes of discovering something new (or at least something entertaining). Sometimes, however, your web experience might be more complex than this. You might, for example, use the Web to manage your e-mail accounts or you might order a book or a CD from on online retailer. In this case, the server is doing something more complex than simply "serving" you the same old HTML files that it serves everyone. It might, for example, be storing your shipping address or tracking items you've purchased in the past in order to make recommendations for other products you might enjoy. The pages you see in these cases are typically created "on the fly," just for you.

In short, the server can be used to perform a number of tasks that make a user's web experience highly dynamic and interactive. In this book, I'm going to show you how to make the server behave in these dynamic ways. Therefore, it is necessary to introduce some useful server-specific terminology right from the get-go. What enables interactivity are programs the server "runs" *CGI scripts*. "CGI" is an acronym for *common gateway interface*, a method or *protocol* by which the server interacts with other software on the server (e.g., databases), as well as with other computers on the Web. There are a number of programs and programming languages that can be used for CGI programming (e.g., Cold Fusion, PHP, ASP, C++). In this book, we're going to focus on Perl. Perl (practical extraction and report language) is a highly versatile programming language and it is one of the most popular languages for CGI scripting.

There is one final distinction that I should make because it will help you better understand how the things we'll be doing fit into the broader Internet context. In this book we'll be focusing on *server-side* programming—writing CGI programs that run on the server. *Client-side* programming, in contrast, involves writing programs that run on the user's (sometimes called the *client's*) browser. You've probably heard of some common client-side programming languages before, such as JavaScript. *JavaScript* is a special kind of code that can be embedded in an HTML document. When the HTML document (a file, actually) is delivered to the user's browser, the JavaScript program is executed by the browser and all the relevant computations (e.g., tallying up a total price) are performed by the user's computer. The advantage of using JavaScript is that, because the computation is done by the user's computer, the server is freed from having to perform resource-consuming functions for multiple users at once. The downside of JavaScript is that different browsers do not always interpret JavaScript code in the same way. (In fact, different versions of the same browser do not even interpret JavaScript code in the same manner!) Sometimes you might need to write separate JavaScript programs depending on whether the user is working with Netscape Navigator or Internet Explorer. Moreover, some users have the JavaScript option turned off on their browser. Most importantly, it is difficult to use JavaScript to save data, making it virtually useless for serious research purposes. Having worked with both server-side and client-side programs, I believe that server-side programming is better suited for the needs of the behavioral scientist.

HOW TO GET THE MOST OUT OF THIS BOOK

In Chapter 2 I will show you how to get a web server up and running. We'll discuss two different ways for getting access to a web server and you will need to chose which method is best for you. One approach is to transform a spare PC into a web server. This is much easier than it may sound, and I'll walk you through each step to help ensure that the process goes smoothly for you. One of the advantages of this approach is that, if you have a spare PC, transforming the computer into a server is cost-free. Another approach is to find a professional web hosting service and use their web server for your research. It is possible that your university or department has a server that can be used for research purposes, but, if not, there are many professional web hosting companies that will allow you to build your research web pages on their computers either free of charge (if you agree to allow the company to display small advertisements on your web pages) or for a trivial fee (e.g., anywhere from $5 to $20 a month, depending on your needs). The primary advantage of this approach is that it will require no server maintenance on your part. In fact, if you have the extra money to spend, I would strongly recommend this approach for the beginner. I would encourage you to skim through Chapter 2, decide which approach seems best suited to your needs, and then follow the steps for that method in order to get your server up and running.

After you successfully set up your server in Chapter 2, I encourage you *to work through each example* as you read the chapters. Learning to write programs is kind of like learning to drive a car. You can read *Driving for Dummies* and become quite knowledgeable about stick shifts and parallel parking, but you won't acquire the necessary skills until you start to get behind the wheel. Designing web experiments is a skill, and your ability to perform the skill well will depend less on memorizing the right kinds of facts and details, which you can look up in a reference manual anyway, and more on acquiring a certain degree of familiarity and intuition concerning the "logic" of programming. Therefore, this book is a "beginner's guide" not because it explains easy tasks, but because I have done my best to walk you through a highly complex terrain without assuming you know your way around. With some practice, you'll come to know this terrain well.

A structured way to use this book would be to work through one chapter a day. As you read each chapter, you should enter the programming code and see the result of the code on an actual web browser, such as Microsoft's Internet Explorer. To make this easy for you, all of the code that is presented in this book can be copied-and-pasted from the website for this book: http://www.web-research-design.net. Moreover, "live" demonstrations of the various studies and applications that we discuss can be accessed at that site. Be sure to tinker with the code a bit and see if things change in the way you expect. Finally, after working your way though a chapter, it might be a good idea to take a break and then reread the chapter. It is easy to lose sight of the "big picture" when you're focusing on the minutia of programming code.

At the end of each chapter I have included, where relevant, a table that contains all of the new HTML or CGI/Perl code that was introduced in that chapter. As you'll observe from thumbing through the book, I introduce the majority of the programming code early in the book, in Chapters 3 through 7. In fact, the latter half of the book uses very little new code. One of the things you'll discover as you begin to learn HTML and Perl is that you don't need to know much in order to accomplish a lot. Many of the complex techniques that we'll discuss later in the book, such as tracking a user's responses over multiple sessions, involve finding novel and creative ways to use the code you already know rather than learning new commands. With this in mind, as you read the book I encourage you to think outside the box and try to envision some of the ways in which the skills you are learning could be reconfigured to address research scenarios not discussed here.

On the website for this book I have created some online quizzes that you can take to test your learning. These quizzes, which are discussed in detail in Chapter 14, will automatically score your answers and give you feedback on your performance. Unlike the quizzes described in Chapter 14, however, they will not tell you the correct answer when you get a question wrong. At the end of each chapter, you may want to take the corresponding quiz a few times until you get it right.

With the exception of Chapter 15, I have deliberately organized the chapters in a manner that will allow you to build on skills that you have acquired earlier in the book. Thus, I recommend that you read through the chapters *sequentially*. Even if you're not interested in randomly assigning participants to different conditions (Chapter 8), the skills covered in that chapter will be critical to understanding things that may be of interest to you in later chapters. It may seem that you can pick and choose among the chapters in this book, but I strongly discourage you from approaching the book in that manner. I have written the chapters in a fashion that allows you to gradually build your programming skills, so you should tackle each chapter in turn—even if it focuses on a research technique that seems tangential to your interests.

I have adopted a few conventions in the book that should make your reading and programming experience easier. First, all code, whether it be HTML or Perl code, will be printed in `Courier typeface`. Labels in the left margin identify the code for the files that are downloadable from http://www.web-research-design.net. **Buttons** and hyperlinks have been set off as shown, and a third category which represents miscellaneous items such as commands, folder names, dialog box names, and so on has been set off. Finally, I have made parenthetical comments or important qualifications throughout the text. Instead of placing these in footnotes (where they would be easily overlooked), I have set them off as Notes and Tips.

Chapter 2

Getting Started

A Step-by-Step Guide to Using a Web Server

Now that you have some background information and know a bit of what to expect, let's get started. In the last chapter you learned that when you visit a web page your computer is requesting information from another computer (i.e., a server) located at that address. That computer "serves" your computer the information you've requested, and your computer's browser renders the information (typically HTML code) in the form of web page. In order to conduct research over the Internet, you will need to find a computer that you can use as a server—a computer that will receive requests, process and manage data, and send new files to your users or research participants.

In this chapter I will show you two alternative methods for getting access to a web server. The first method we will discuss involves using a professional web hosting service. One of the advantages of this approach is that the web hosting company will provide, house, and maintain the server. All you need to do is write your HTML and CGI programs on your own computer and transfer the files to the server via file transfer programs. (I'll explain what a file transfer program is later, but, for now, think of this process as akin to e-mailing your documents to someone else.) If the web hosting company you choose offers its services for free, the company will probably cover its costs by placing ads on your web page. Or, you might choose a fee-based hosting service and avoid the ads. In this chapter I'll show you how to set up a server for free with a web hosting company called Netfirms.

The second method we will discuss involves setting up a server of your own. Specifically, I will show you how to transform a spare PC into a fully functioning web server. The advantage to having your own web server is that you can store as much information on the server as the computer is capable of holding. In contrast, if you use a web hosting company, the company will place limits on the amount of space that you can use on their server. Another advantage of using your own server is you will not have to use file transfer programs to transfer the programs that you write from your computer to the server. If you create all the programs *on* your server, there is no need to transfer anything. One of the disadvantages of setting up your own server is that having a server requires some degree of maintenance on your part. As will be discussed in Chapter 15, you will need to periodically reboot the machine when things go wrong, make sure it doesn't get turned off by accident, and rotate various log files (i.e., files that keep track of errors, web access). In short, using your own server, while having its advantages, can be a high maintenance approach to conducting research over the Internet.

Which of these two approaches should you use? Relatively inexperienced computer users will probably find it easier to use a web hosting service. If you're feeling a bit more adventurous, don't want to pay service fees, or want more control over what you can do with your server, you should consider setting up your own personal server. I'll discuss both methods in this chapter. If you're not completely sure which method you want to pursue at this point, I would encourage you to skim the remainder of this chapter to get a sense for what is involved with these two approaches. You may discover, for example, that it is unfeasible for you to setup your own server (e.g., you might not have a spare computer for this purpose). So, give the chapter a skim, choose a method that seems best suited to your needs and resources, then work systematically through the steps corresponding to that method. You will probably find this chapter a bit challenging if you're not used to downloading and installing programs, but once you've accomplished these basic tasks, you will be rewarded with a fully operational web server!

METHOD 1: USING A PROFESSIONAL WEB HOSTING SERVICE

In this section I will show you how to set up a server with a professional web hosting company named Netfirms (http://www.netfirms.com/). I have chosen this particular company because I have researched them thoroughly and believe that **Netfirms** offers the services best suited to our needs for a fair price—starting with the low, low price of $0. Of course, Netfirms is not the only company you could use, but I have chosen it in order to be able to focus on one hosting service in particular. I want to make sure I can walk you through the techniques covered in this book with no ambiguities. If I were to describe the *general* process of using a web hosting service without showing you how to use one service in particular, you would be forced to navigate the idiosyncrasies of various hosting services alone. Once you've mastered the techniques in covered in this book, you will know enough to adapt your skills to servers provided by other hosting companies. (Later in this chapter I'll provide some tips and guidelines for those who are adventurous enough to try an alternative hosting service.) For our purposes, the most important features of Netfirms are as follows

- Netfirms provides a free web hosting service. Signing up takes less than 5 minutes, and your account is activated within minutes.
- Both their free and paid services allow you to use Perl and CGI scripts. This is critical because very few free web hosting services will allow you to use your own CGI scripts.
- Although Netfirms is able to provide you with free hosting by placing ads on your web pages, you can upgrade your service for a nominal fee. Importantly, you can upgrade with Netfirms easily and without having to restructure your server or your files. With a few simple mouse clicks, the ads will be gone.

If you choose to use a hosting company other than Netfirms, make sure that the company will allow you to post your own CGI scripts. Some companies will offer you CGI capabilities, but, if you read the fine print, you'll discover that you can only run CGI programs that the company provides, not scripts that you have written. You will also want to find out exactly what their advertising policy is and how easy it will be to remove the advertisements if you decide to upgrade your service.

Signing Up with Netfirms

To get started, go to the main web page for Netfirms: http://www.netfirms. com. Near the lower left of the page you should see a link that says "Free Web Hosting" When you click that link, you will be taken to a page that explains what Netfirms provides for free. Click on the button that says "signup now." The first thing you will need to do is choose a **domain name**. A domain name is kind of like a business name for your site. The domain name for this book's website is web-research-design and the corresponding URL is http://www. web-research-design.net/. You can choose either to create a personalized domain name (e.g., web-research-design) for approximately $25 a year or a free domain name if you are willing to allow your site's address to be a "sub-domain" of Netfirms (e.g., webbook.netfirms.com).

For the purposes of illustrating the registration process, I have registered a free account at Netfirms using their free domain name option. The sub-domain name is "webbook" and the full URL for my free site is http://www. webbook.netfirms.com. For now, you may want to choose the free option; you can always upgrade your account and obtain a personal domain name at a later time. To take the free route, click the link I prefer a free Netfirms Subdomain, enter the name you would like to use, and click **Search**. If that name has not been chosen by someone else, you will be allowed to proceed to the next step. If that name has been used already, Netfirms will ask you to try submitting another name.

In Step 3 you will review your order. Click the **Continue** button, unless you want to upgrade your service. Next you will need to enter your mailing address. After completing this information make sure you agree to Netfirms' Terms of Service by clincking on that link, and then on the internal link on that page, Netfirms Basic Hosting Plan Additional Terms. Then, return to the contact info page, click the box next to I have read, understood and accepted the Netfirms Terms of Service, and press the **Continue** button. In Step 4 you will verify this information and press the **Continue** button.

Once you click the **Continue** button you will be taken to a new page that informs you that your registration is complete. Netfirms will e-mail you the information you will need, such as your password. Once you receive this e-mail, which should be within minutes, you'll be ready to customize your website.

Transferring Files to Your Netfirms Server

Because the Netfirms server is not located in the same place as you, you will need a way to transfer the HTML and CGI programs that you write on your computer to the Netfirms server. To do so, you will need a **File Transfer Protocol** (FTP) program for your computer. In this chapter I will show you how to use a FTP program called **WS_FTP Pro**—one of the most commonly used file transfer programs available.

WS_FTP Pro is a commercial program. The instructions below show how to download a free evaluation version of the program, but the evaluation version will be good for only 30 days. After 30 days, you'll need to purchase the program. If you are a student or faculty member at a university, however, there is a high likelihood that you already have an FTP program, such as WS FTP, installed on your computer. (To check whether you already have a copy, simply click on your **Start** button, move your mouse to Find and Files or folders and conduct a search for *ftp*.exe. Be sure to include the asterisks; the asterisks instruct Windows to search for any file name that contains "ftp.") If you do not have a version of WS_FTP or another FTP program on your computer, it is highly likely that you can obtain a free "educational version" from your university's computing center. In the meantime, go ahead and download the evaluation copy; you can check with your university's computer center at a later time.

If you have used an FTP program in the past and feel comfortable with it, there will be no need to follow the installation notes below, and you can skip ahead to the configuration section where I show you how to FTP to your space on the Netfirms server.

Downloading and Installing WS_FTP Pro

1. Go to the Downloads, Evaluation Software page for WS_FTP Pro at http://www.ipswitch.com/Products/WS_FTP/.

2. A new page will appear that shows which kinds of FTP programs you can download. Select the English trial version of WS_FTP Pro.

3. Fill out a short info gathering page, and click **Submit**.

4. You will now be given the option to download WS_FTP Pro from a number of websites. Choose the site that is geographically closest to you and click its link.

5. A File Download window will open. Choose the **Save this file to disk** option, and save the file to your Desktop. At the time of this writing (July 2003), the file name was called f_x86t32.exe.

6. Once you've downloaded the file, double click the f_x86t32.exe icon on your Desktop.

7. An Installation Wizard should appear. Follow the instructions and, unless you're experienced and confident with computers, choose all the defaults. Once the installation is complete (this may take several minutes), you'll be given the option to run the FTP program. For now, close the program. Notice that there is a new icon on your Desktop labeled WS_FTP Pro. You will double-click this icon whenever you want to use your file transfer program.

Configuring WS_FTP Pro

Before you can use your file transfer program to move files back and forth between your computer and your Netfirms server, you'll need to configure WS_FTP Pro so that it knows which server you want to exchange files with. You'll only need to configure WS_FTP Pro once.

1. Double click the WS_FTP Pro icon on your desktop.

2. Chose the **Start Evaluation** button.

3. If the Connect to Remote Host window does not pop up, click the button at the lower left labeled **Connect**.

4. The Connect to Run of a Host window will appear. Chose the **Create Site** option.

5. A new window will appear asking you for a **Profile Name**. A Profile Name is simply a nickname of sorts—something that allows *you* to keep track of the various FTP connections you may want to establish. Chose something simple, such as "my server" and click the **Next** button.

6. Next you will need to provide the Host Address for the server to which you would like to connect. This information will be provided in the e-mail that Netfirms has sent you. Look for the line in that e-mail that starts with "FTP server name" or "FTP Address." Enter that name in the box provided and click **Next**. For my free account, the host address is webbook.netfirms.com.

7. Next you will need to enter your Login Credentials. In short, this is your Username or Membername, which you will put into the User ID box, and Password. This information will also have been provided in the e-mail you received from Netfirms. It is okay to leave the Account box empty. Press the **Finish** button.

> **Note.** The WS_FTP Pro software is updated on a fairly regular basis. However, the configuration steps that I've described above should be fairly general from one version to the next. The critical things to be entered are (1) the Profile Name (e.g., "my server"), (2) the host (i.e., the computer or server with which you wish to transfer files, such as yourname. netfirms.com), and (3) your **Username** (e.g., yourname) and **Password**. There will often be other options (e.g., a checkbox for **Anonymous** or **Account Information**) that you can leave empty.

Using WS_FTP Pro to Transfer Files

You will be using WS_FTP Pro to transfer files from your computer to the server at Netfirms. You can also transfer files from your Netfirms server to your computer. Unfortunately, if you're new to the file transfer process, you'll probably find it a bit difficult to understand at first. With some hands-on experience, however, you'll become adept in no time. When I was first learning to use an FTP program, I found it useful to conceptualize the program as an interface that allowed me to treat the server as if it were a disk drive. For example, if I want to copy a file on my hard drive to a floppy disk I simply find the file on my hard drive (using an application such as My Computer or

Windows Explorer) and copy it to the floppy. Similarly, if I wanted to take a file on my floppy disk and transfer it to my hard drive, I simply find the file on my floppy disk and send it to the hard drive. WS_FTP Pro works the same way—it provides you with a virtual disk drive for your Netfirms server so that you can transfer files between your computer and the server. I'll expand a bit on this analogy below, but let's first get the program running so you can see how to use it.

1. Double click on the WS_FTP Pro icon on your Desktop.

2. When the program loads, you may need to click on a **Begin Evaluation** or **Continue Evaluation** button if the program is not registered. Go ahead and click that button.

3. Click on the Profile Name (e.g., "my server") and click **Connect**.

4. You should now see two directory windows (see Figure 2.1). The window on the left-hand side displays the directory structure for *your* computer. This is often called the Local directory window. This window works in the same way as the directory windows that you use when you click on the My Computer icon on your Desktop or when you're opening or saving a file in a program such as Microsoft Word. In the example in Figure 2.1, you can see that I'm currently situated in the C:\Program Files\WS_FTP Pro directory and the window displays all the folders and files located in that directory. I can move "backwards" or "higher up" in the directory structure by clicking the icon that looks like a folder with an "up" arrow. I will refer to this icon as the **Up Button** throughout this chapter. If I want to move "down" or "forward" in the directory structure, I can simply click on the folder I wish to open. In short, to move forward through the directory structure, click the folder you wish to open; to move backward through the structure, click the **Up Button**.

The window on the right-hand side contains the directory structure of your Netfirms server. This is often called the Remote directory window because it contains the directory structure for a computer other than the one at which you're currently sitting (i.e., one at a remote location). You should see three folders, one called admin, one called cgi-bin, and one called www. You will not be able to access the admin

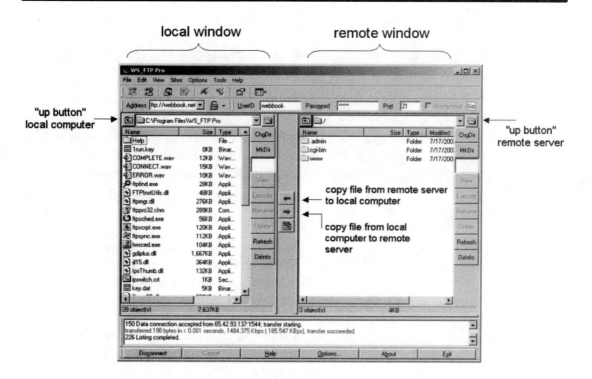

FIGURE 2.1. WS_FTP Pro layout.

folder, so ignore that folder. The other two folders are critical. You will be using the **www** folder to hold the HTML web pages that you create and the **cgi-bin** folder to hold any CGI/Perl programs that you create. I'll explain the function of these two folders in more depth later. For now, notice that you can open the **www** folder, for example, by double-clicking on it. To move out of this folder, simply click the **Up Button** corresponding to the remote directory window (see Figure 2.1).

As you can see, WS_FTP Pro provides you with two directory structures, side by side. The window on the left displays the directory structure for your computer; the window on the right displays the directory structure for your Netfirms server. If I wish to transfer a file from my computer to the server, I find the file in my local directory structure, select the file of interest so as to highlight it, and then click the button with the green, left-to-right arrow in between the two windows (see Figure 2.1). This instructs the program to take the file on my computer and "shoot it over" or copy it to the server. Similarly, if I want to transfer a file from the server to my computer, I click the file in the remote window to highlight it and click the green right-to-left arrow to transfer it to the local window.

It is important to keep in mind that the file transfer process is conceptually identical to copying a file from your hard drive to a floppy or vice versa. In both cases, we are doing nothing more than moving a copy of a file from one location to another location. One of the common mistakes that beginners make is they assume that, if they change or edit an HTML or CGI file on their computer, the changes will immediately be reflected on the server. It doesn't work this way. Please keep the floppy disk analogy in mind. Imagine creating a Microsoft Word document on your computer and saving it to floppy disk. If you were to mail the disk to a colleague, but later decide to delete a few paragraphs from the file on your computer, your colleague will still have the copy with those paragraphs. If you want to change or update an HTML file, you'll need to transfer the updated file from your local computer to the server in order for web users to see the revised document.

Creating a Data Directory

As you'll discover later in this book, some of the programs that we will write will collect data from our users and save those data to the server. We will want to create a special directory in which to save our data files so that we don't mix them up with our other files.

1. Given the way Netfirms configures its server, we will need to place our new data folder within the www folder. To open the www folder, double click on it.

2. Click on the **MkDir** button on the remote window to make a new directory.

3. When the Make directory window appears, type in, "data" (without the quotes) and press the **OK** button.

You should now have a new directory called **data** that is embedded within the **www** directory. Make sure you're comfortable moving into and out of this directory. When you establish an FTP connection for the first time after creating this directory, you'll need to double-click the **www** folder in order to see the **data** folder. Then, to open the **data** folder, you'll need to double-click on it. To move backwards or out of the folder, simply click the **Up Button**.

Some Important Notes on the Organization and Operation of Your Server

The Location of Your Web Pages

As mentioned previously, your Netfirms server has two folders of interest: the **cgi-bin** folder and the **www** folder. The **www** folder is what is sometimes called a **Public HTML** folder because its contents can be viewed by anyone surfing the Web. When we begin creating web pages in Chapter 3, we will be placing those HTML pages into your **Public HTML** folder so that other people can view them.

> **Note.** Whenever you create a standard **HTML** web page in this book, I will ask you to save it to the **www** folder on your Netfirms server. In the remainder of this book, I will refer to this folder or directory as the **Public HTML** folder, therefore, when I ask you to save a file to the **Public HTML** folder, I mean to transfer it to the **www** folder in your Netfirms account.

The Address or URL for Your Web Page

The full URL for your website should be included in the e-mail that you received from Netfirms. In the example above, the URL for the free website that I've created is http://webbook.netfirms.com/, and this URL will be part of the address for any web page I create. If I created a web page called **MemoryStudy.htm** and saved it to my **Public HTML** folder, the address for that page would be http://webbook.netfirms.com/MemoryStudy.htm.

The CGI Folder

As was discussed in Chapter 1, we'll be writing CGI scripts in order to do special things, such as store our data. Unlike HTML files (i.e., your standard web pages), these files will be *executable* programs, and they will be stored in the special folder called cgi-bin. When you write a CGI program, you will *always* save it to the cgi-bin directory on your Netfirms account.

> **Note.** Whenever you create a **CGI script**, you will save it to the cgi-bin directory on your server. I will refer to this directory as the cgi-bin directory for the remainder of this book.

Transferring Files

Throughout this book I will ask you to create new HTML and CGI files and save them to your server. Please keep in mind that you will need to save the file to your local computer first and then transfer it to the appropriate folder on your server using your FTP program. If I ask you to save a file as example1.htm in your Public HTML folder, you should (1) save the file as example1.htm somewhere on your computer (e.g., on your Desktop or My Documents folder), (2) open your FTP program and establish a connection with the server, and (3) transfer the file example1.htm from your computer to the Public HTML folder on the server. If I ask you to save a file as perlscript.pl in your server's cgi-bin, you should (1) save the file as perlscript.pl somewhere on your computer (e.g., on your Desktop or My Documents folder), (2) open your FTP program and establish a connection with the server, and (3) transfer the file perlscript.pl from your computer to the cgi-bin folder on your server. *If you are using a web hosting service such as Netfirms you will need to follow this general procedure for all the examples discussed in this book.*

Timing Out

For security purposes, many web hosting companies will automatically end your FTP connection if there isn't any file transfer activity within a certain period of time (e.g., 3 minutes). If this happens to you, simply restart the FTP process by clicking the **Close** button and then the **Connect** button.

METHOD 2: SETTING UP YOUR OWN SERVER

In this section I will show you how to set up your own server if you are not interested in using a professional web hosting company. The first thing you'll need to do is find a computer that you can use for this purpose. If you have a spare PC in your lab that runs Windows 95/98/2000/ME/XP and has a high-speed Internet connection, it should do the trick. If you only have one computer (e.g., your office computer), you can use it as a server while still using it for your normal day-to-day activities. However, as you might expect, the more activities you have your computer doing at one time, the slower it will run. If you have a computer that was purchased sometime after 1998, this probably won't have a noticeable impact on your day-to-day work, unless you do a lot of computational simulations or tend to download large files.

First, make sure your future server is on and connected to the Internet. You'll want to make sure that your future server has a **static IP address**. Having, a static IP address means that there is a specific—and unchanging—numeric code associated with your computer. This code needs to be unchanging if your computer is going to be used as a server. If you are using your computer from home and use AOL or SBC, for example, as your Internet service provider, chances are that you have what is called a **dynamic IP address**. If so, the IP address associated with your computer will change every time you log onto the Web. You will need an unchanging IP address if people are going to be able to request web pages from your server reliably. (As an analogy, a static IP address is like a permanent mailing address and a dynamic IP address is a bit like a temporary post office box number.) You may request a static IP address from your Internet service provider for a home computer, but doing so may cost a little bit extra. If you are working with a university or office computer, there is a high probability that your computer has a static IP address. But, if you have any doubts, please contact your department's information technology associate. Depending on how the department's computer network is organized, it may or may not be feasible for you to configure your own server.

If your computer is configured to run "scheduled checks" at various times of the day or week, please turn those options off. Once your server is functional, you'll probably want to leave it on 24 hours a day during periods when you're collecting data. If your computer is defragmenting the hard drive while users are trying to understand their personality things will get wacky pretty quickly. If you have an anti-virus program that scans or filters incoming data and mail, leave that on. However, make sure your computer is not scheduled to do scans of your entire hard drive on a regular basis. If you want to perform such scans, find a low-use time when you can turn your server off and perform the scan manually.

Before your computer can operate as a web server, we'll need to download the appropriate software. We're going to download three programs: Microsoft Installer, ActiveState Perl, and Apache server software. I'll explain the purpose of these programs below as I show you how to download them.

Downloading and Installing Microsoft's Windows Installer

Open up an Internet connection using your favorite browser, such as Microsoft's Internet Explorer or Netscape's Navigator.

> **Note.** The steps I describe here were appropriate in July 2003. It may be the case that new versions of these programs have been released in the meantime. If this appears to be the case, simply download the most recent versions and keep in mind that some of the steps may have changed as a consequence. As I become aware of significant changes in the process described below, I'll keep the changes posted on the book's website: http://www.web-research-design.net/.

Microsoft's Windows Installer is a program that will facilitate the installation of some of the other programs that you'll be downloading. If you have Windows 2000 or XP, you will not need to download this program and you should skip to the next section on ActivePerl. If you have Windows 95/98/ Me, you'll need to download Windows Installer.

1. Go to the following website: http://www.activestate.com. This is also the site from which we'll download ActivePerl (or Perl). Fortunately, Perl can be easily installed with the assistance of Microsoft's Windows Installer, so we'll download that program first.

2. Find the link on the page labeled <u>Downloads</u>. Click on the smaller <u>download</u> link that goes with the <u>ActivePerl</u> link.

3. Clicking this link will bring you to a page that asks for your e-mail address so that you may receive updates. Technically, you don't need to register to download ActivePerl. I have registered, however, and, to the

best of my knowledge, I've never received unwanted e-mail as a consequence of doing so. Once you've registered (or decided not to register), click on the **Next** button at the bottom of the page.

4. The next page explains the system requirements for ActivePerl. There is a link on this page for downloading Windows Installer. (As of July 2003, the area containing the link was in a gray box on the right-hand side of the page in a section that gives options for downloading **Windows Installer 2.0+**.) Click on the Windows Installer link appropriate for your Windows system to download the installer program. (Unless you're using Windows NT, select the link that says <u>download for 9x/Me</u>. If you don't know which version of Windows you're running, click on the **Help** menu of Windows Explorer or My Computer, and then the **About Windows . . .** choice at the bottom of the menu will tell you.)

5. Once you've clicked the Windows Installer link, a **File Download** window should appear. Select the **Save this program to disk** option and click **OK**. For simplicity, I recommend that you save this, and other programs we'll download, to your **Desktop**. At the time of this writing, the Windows Installer file was called **InstMsiA.exe**.

6. Once the file has downloaded successfully, you should be able to find an icon labeled **InstMsiA.exe** on your desktop. Double-click on that icon in order to install the program.

7. If you have any other programs open, the installer program will probably ask you to close them. Once the program has successfully installed, you'll need to restart your computer.

Downloading and Installing ActivePerl

ActivePerl is a package that we can download for free that contains Perl and some other useful resources. As discussed previously, Perl is the programming language we'll be using for our CGI scripting. The aspects of the language we'll be using are not too complex, and we'll work with many examples in order to illustrate how the code operates. In fact, you'll probably be able to tailor many of the examples we discuss in this book to suit your needs without having to do much programming on your own. We can download ActivePerl from the ActiveState website.

1. Return to the ActiveState website at http://www.activestate.com, and go back to the screen we were at when we downloaded the Windows Installer (see the instructions above).

2. You'll now have the option to download ActivePerl for several systems (e.g., Windows, Linux). Since the package is updated fairly regularly, you may see several different versions—sometimes called "builds." Find the version with the highest build number. (At the time of this writing, the highest build or version was numbered 806.) Click on the option for Windows labeled <u>MSI</u>. This will allow you to download a version of ActivePerl that can be installed easily using Microsoft's Windows Installer.

3. Again, a File Download window will open. Choose the **Save this file to disk** option, and save the file (ActivePerl-5.8.0.806-MSWin32-x86.msi) to your Desktop.

4. Once you've downloaded the file, double click the ActivePerl-5.8.0. 806-MSWin32-x86 icon on your desktop.

5. An Installation Wizard should appear. Please follow all the instructions, and *choose all the defaults*. (The only exception to this rule concerns the license for the software. Be sure to *accept* the terms of the agreement [which is not the default option]. If you do not accept their terms, the installation process will abort.) Once the installation is complete (this may take several minutes), you'll need to restart your computer.

Downloading and Installing the Apache Server

We'll be using the term *server* throughout this book to refer to both the software that performs server functions, as well as the server computer. Since you've already designated a computer as your physical server, we now need to download the software it needs to behave like one.

Apache is one of the most widely used server programs. It is based on **open-source** code, which means that the software has been developed by independent programmers and development teams who believe that important, building-block software should be freely available; it is not a commercial venture. Periodically, the most efficient version of the code is modified or updated on the basis of new developments, and posted for free download at the Apache Software Foundation website.

1. Go to the Apache website at http://www.apache.org/.

2. Click on the HTTP Server link under the Apache Projects heading/ link on the left.

3. Find the Download! section. At the time of this writing there is only one link labeled from a mirror. Click that link. (A "mirror" is a site other than the current site that holds the software you intend to download).

4. The download page ought to have a section that tells you which version of Apache is the most stable and current version. At the time of this writing, the section was titled Apache 2.0.47 is the best available version. Within this section there are several files that can be downloaded. Chose the link for Win32 Binary (MSI Installer). At the time of this writing, the linked filename was apache_2.0.47-win32-x86-no_ssl.msi.

5. A File Download window should open. Save the file apache_2.0.47-win32-x86-no_ssl.msi to your Desktop. As improved versions of Apache are created and posted, some (minor) aspects of my instructions may no longer apply. If something seems to have changed by the time you read this, all you need to do is determine which version of Apache is the most stable (this will be noted clearly on the Apache website), and download the *Win32 binary* version with a .msi extension so that the Windows Installer program can install it.

6. Once the file is downloaded, double-click on the corresponding icon on your Desktop. This should open an Apache Installation Wizard window. Follow all the instructions, and *go with the defaults*. One of the windows, depicted in the Figure 2.2, is important. You'll want to write down *all* the pertinent information. The Server Name box, for example, contains the URL for your future website. As can be seen in Figure 2.2, I'm installing my Apache server on a computer whose URL will be http://P032.psch.uic.edu.

   Each of these boxes should have something filled in automatically by the installation program. If so, please do not change anything except the contents of the box labeled Administrator's Email Address.

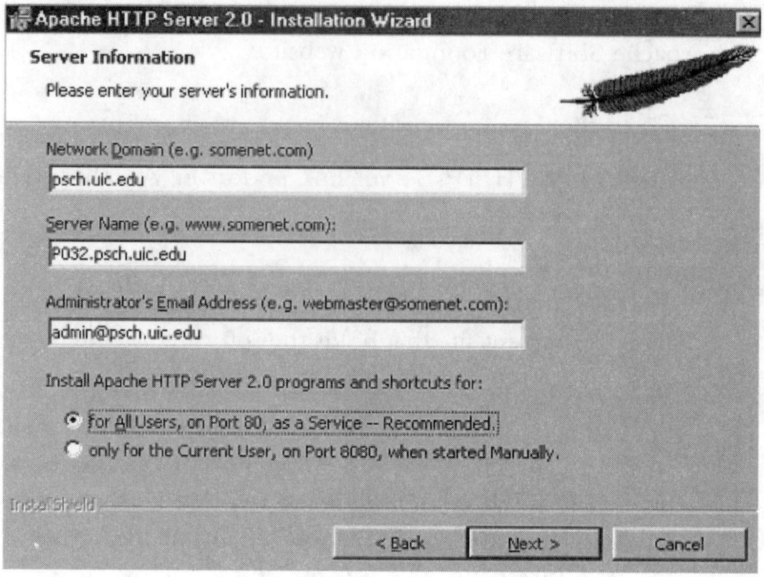

FIGURE 2.2. Apache installation wizard window.

You should type your e-mail address in that box. If these boxes are empty, cancel the installation process and consult the Troubleshooting section toward the end of this chapter.

7. Once the program has installed successfully, you'll need to restart your computer.

Getting Your Server Up and Running

Now that you have downloaded and installed all the programs you need, you're ready to set up and test your server.

1. Go to your Windows **Start** menu and click on the following sequence of options: Programs > Apache HTTP Server > Control Apache Server > Start Apache in Console. This will open an MS-DOS window. *Do not close this window.* It is okay to minimize it, but do not close it. It needs to be open in order for the server software to be operational.

2. Let's test Apache. Open your browser and enter the following URL: http://localhost.

3. If you've been successful, you'll see the page depicted in Figure 2.3. If you see this page, you should celebrate. Why? Earlier today you were skeptical over whether you'd be conducting your own Internet research within a couple of days, now you have your own, fully operational server. Congratulations!

If you don't see a page similar to that illustrated in Figure 2.3, please retrace your steps and make sure everything was done correctly. It is easy to overlook a simple step in the installation process. For example, you may have downloaded the wrong file (e.g., a source file rather than a binary). If you can't correct the problem, please consult the Troubleshooting section of this chapter. I will keep an up-to-date Frequently Asked Questions page, as well as a troubleshooting page, on the website for this book.

Creating a Data Directory

As you'll discover later in this book, some of the programs we will write will collect data from our users and save those data to the server. It is customary to create a special directory in which to save our data files so that we don't mix them up with our other files. There are a number of places where you can place this folder if you're using your own server. However, in order to ensure that the programming code used in this book is compatible with your server, you'll need to create a specific directory.

1. Use your **My Computer** application on your desktop to locate the C:\Program Files\Apache Group\Apache2\htdocs\ directory.

2. Within that htdocs folder, create a new folder called www.

3. Within the new www folder, create an additional folder called data.

In the programs we discuss later in this book, we will be collecting data from participants and those programs will automatically store those data in the following directory: C:\Program Files\Apache Group\Apache2\htdocs\ www\data. As I'll explain in Chapter 5, you can access that data on your

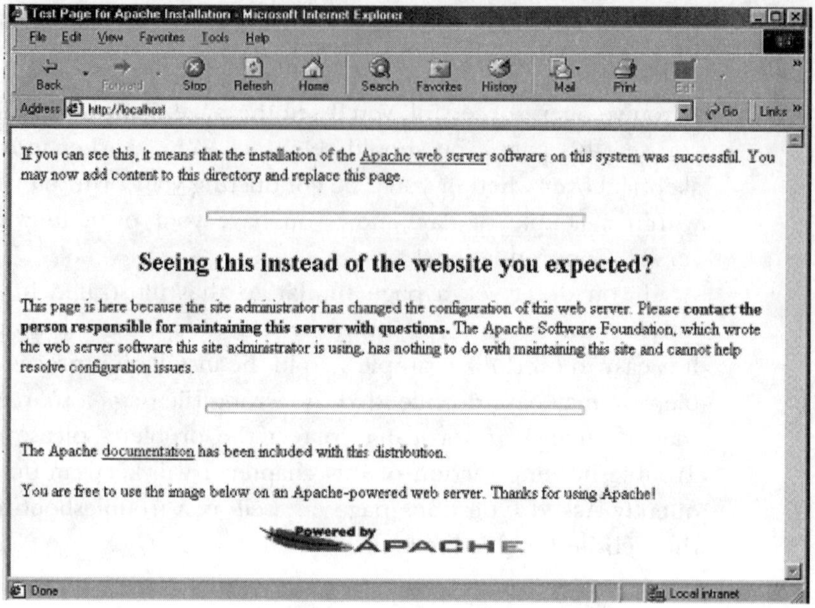

FIGURE 2.3. You should see this screen if you have successfully installed the Apache server software.

server by simply going to this folder. In Chapter 15 I'll show you an alternative way of configuring your **data** folder that will keep its contents more secure, but this approach will be easiest for learning the skills taught in this book.

Some Important Notes about the Organization and Operation of Your Server

Transferring Files to the Server

If you've created web pages in the past, but didn't have your own server, you're probably familiar with **File Transfer Protocol** (**FTP**) programs, such as

WS_FTP Pro. FTP programs are used to transfer documents from one computer to another via the Internet. Now that you have your own server, you will *not* need to use an FTP program. You can create your programs on the server itself, and, since they are already on the server, you won't need to transfer them there. This will make the process quicker and more gratifying.

The Location of Your Web Pages

Although your computer is now functioning as a server, it is not the case that all of the directories and files on your computer are available for people to see. Only files in the specific folder htdocs can be viewed by people visiting your website. If you followed all the defaults when installing Apache, this folder should be located in the following directory: C:\Program Files\Apache Group\Apache2\htdocs\. Once you create an HTML document and place it in this folder, it can be viewed by anyone else in the world who types in the correct URL. If you created and saved the document in, let's say, the My Documents folder, it would *not* be viewable by others.

> **Note.** Whenever you create a standard **HTML** web page, you will save it to the C:\Program Files\Apache Group\Apache2\htdocs\ directory on your server. In the remainder of this book, I will refer to this folder or directory as the **Public HTML** folder. If I ask you to save a file to your **Public HTML folder**, you should save it to the C:\Program Files\Apache Group\ Apache2\htdocs\ folder on your web server.

The Address or URL for Your Web Pages

Recall the **Server Name** box that appeared when we were installing Apache? The name that appeared in that box is the "base" or "root" URL for your site (i.e., the URL for all pages on your site will begin with that root). So let's say I have created a web page called MemoryStudy.htm and saved it in my Public HTML folder. The full URL for that page would be http://P032.psch.uic. edu/MemoryStudy.htm. Anyone typing http://P032.psch.uic.edu/MemoryStudy. htm into the URL bar on his or her browser will go straight to that web page. (Please note that the 0 in "P032" is a zero, and not the capital letter O.)

The CGI Folder

As we discussed in Chapter 1, we'll be writing CGI scripts in Perl in order to do special things, such as store our data. Unlike HTML files (i.e., your standard web pages), these files will be *executable* programs, and they will be stored in a special folder called cgi-bin. If you followed all the defaults when installing Apache, this folder should be located in the following place: C:\Program Files\Apache Group\Apache2\cgi-bin\. When you write a CGI program in Perl, you will *always* save it to the cgi-bin directory.

> **Note.** Whenever you create a **CGI script**, you will save it to the C:\Program Files\Apache Group\Apache2\cgi-bin\ directory on your server. I will refer to this directory as the **cgi-bin** directory for the remainder of this book.

Turning On and Turning Off the Server

As a general rule, you'll be leaving your computer on at all times. One of the valuable things about collecting data over the Internet is that research participants can participate in your study at all times of the day. If you need to turn off your computer, you'll want to first Shut Down your server. To do so, simply go to the open Apache command window (the MS-DOS window) and click on the X in the upper-right corner (the button typically used to close a window). Your computer may or may not complain about this, but it will be fine. Once you have closed this window, you may turn off your computer.

To restart your server, go to your **Start** menu and select the following sequence of options: **Programs > Apache HTTP Server > Control Apache Server > Start Apache in Console**. As noted before, this will open an **MS-DOS** window which must stay open (although you can minimize it) in order for the server to be operational.

> **Note.** On some Windows operating systems, such as Windows 2000, Apache will automatically be turned on whenever you turn on your computer. If this is the case, a message will appear that tells you that the server is already running if you try the steps above.

Troubleshooting

If you follow the basic steps outlined here, everything should work fine. If something doesn't appear to be working correctly, you may want to retrace your steps and work your way through each step again. I will keep an up-to-date troubleshooting section on the web page for this book at http://www. web-research-design.net in case problems emerge that are not addressed in this chapter.

When I try to install the Apache software, the program does not automatically complete the boxes for my Server Name, and so on.

There are at least two reasons why these boxes may not complete themselves automatically. First, if you are using a computer with an Internet connection that employs a dynamic, as opposed to a static, IP address, the server software will not operate appropriately. Second, if your computer was not fully configured for a specific IP address, it is possible that these boxes will appear empty. This will not be a problem in the long run, but it will make the installation process a little more complex. Please ask your university or departmental computer support to configure your computer's IP address. An **IP** (Internet Protocol) address is a sequence of digits (e.g., 121.23.123.23) that acts as an address or location for your computer on the network. All computers connected to the Internet have an IP address associated with them, but some computers are assigned a different IP address each time the user logs onto the Internet, whereas other computers use the same IP address each time the user logs onto the Internet. (By default, Windows systems are often configured to obtain an IP address automatically under the assumption that you are using your computer at home and that your Internet connection will be dynamically assigned by an Internet Service Provider, such as AOL or Prodigy.)

If your computer is not configured to a specific IP address, Apache may not be able to complete the information in the configuration box. You should ask your department's or university's computer support staff to configure your computer to a specific IP address. Once this is done, try to install Apache. Apache should then complete the boxes automatically. If Apache still does not complete the relevant information but you have the IP address, you can treat the IP address as part of the URL for your server. For example, if your IP number is 121.23.123.23, the full URL for your website will be http://121.23.123.23/ instead of something like http://p032.psch.uic.edu/. If this works, contact your computer support staff about obtaining a URL or domain name that corresponds to this IP number that will be easier to use.

I can't find the server file that I need on the Apache website.

The Apache website is updated frequently, so it is unlikely that the exact steps described in this book for downloading the Apache software will be appropriate for long. In general, however, there is a strategy that you want to follow in order to obtain the correct file. Whenever you go to the main website for Apache, (1) find and click on the link for downloading the software for the HTTP Server, (2) find a link for anything that seems pertinent to Windows, such as "win32" or "win9x," and (3) find a package to download that is recent and stable (the page should indicate which version is the most stable) that has the ".msi" extension. The .msi extension means the Microsoft Windows Installer can install the program.

I downloaded the Apache software with no problems, but when I type http://localhost into my browser's URL bar, I don't see the page I'm supposed to see.

It is possible that you didn't turn on the Apache server, or that you had it on previously, but rebooted your computer and now the server is inactive. To start the Apache program, go to your **Start** menu and, under **Programs** or **Applications**, find the Apache program group and look for an option that says **Start console in window** or **Start** within the **Control Apache Server** subgroup. This should open up an **MS-DOS** window (or a **Command Prompt** window, as the **MS-DOS** program was renamed for Windows 2000 and after). You'll need to leave this window open in order for the server to run.

Chapter 3

HTML

How to Make a Web Page from Scratch

Now that you have an operational server, you're ready to begin creating web pages. web pages are generally coded in a language called **HTML** (HyperText Markup Language), so in this chapter we'll discuss how to create basic HTML pages. Specifically, I'll show you how to create a simple page, format text (i.e., use bold, italics, line breaks), insert images, and use hyperlinks. Once you've mastered these basics, I'll show you some more complex HTML techniques in Chapter 4.

We'll be coding our HTML "by hand." There are a number of programs available, such as Microsoft's FrontPage, Macromedia's Dreamweaver, or Netscape's Composer, that allow you to create a web page as if you were working with a word processing program. For example, if you want to place some text in bold, you simply highlight the text and click on the "bold" button. With these **WYSIWYG** (What You See Is What You Get) programs, the way the page looks on your screen is the way the final product is supposed to appear. The HTML code is automatically created in the background, so you don't need to know anything about HTML to create beautiful web pages.

I do not have anything against WYSIWYG programs, and I often use Dreamweaver to manage most of my personal and teaching-related web pages. However, for research purposes, you will need to code most of your HTML "by hand" for two reasons. First, for much of our CGI scripting, we'll need to create new web pages that are tailored for a specific user or research participant. In order to accomplish this we will need to place *generic* HTML code into our CGI scripts. We simply cannot use a WYSIWYG program to construct the appropriate HTML. Second, WYSIWYG programs often insert a lot of useless, and sometimes troublesome, HTML code into your page. Moreover, as you revise pages over time, many WYSIWYG programs do not update the HTML efficiently. This leads to formatting problems that cannot be corrected without explicit knowledge of HTML. You'll want to have *full* control over the pages you create for research purposes, and these programs will not give you the control you need.

It is easiest to write and edit HTML code in a simple text editor. Although you can use a popular word processing program, such as Microsoft Word, to edit text (.txt) files, it is not unusual for MS Word to reformat your text against your will. Therefore, I discourage you from using MS Word for creating HTML files. I also discourage you from using the standard Windows text editor, Notepad, because it has a nasty habit of adding .txt as an extension to all of your files, even if you instruct the program to save the file using an alternative extension.

In this book, I will encourage you to use a text editor called **1st Page**. This program has several desirable features: (1) you can keep multiple files open at once, and move between them easily by simply clicking a tab; (2) the program is "code smart" and will use different colors for various HTML (and Perl) codes, thereby making editing and troubleshooting much easier; (3) the program includes a preview pane, which allows you to see how your HTML code will appear in a browser; (4) like Dreamweaver, the program will do some of the HTML coding for you via drop-down menus, but in a way that is more easily controlled; and (5) the program includes a useful spell-checker that checks your spelling as you type (much like Microsoft Word's). In the next section I will show you how to download and install a free copy of 1st Page. If you have an alternative text editor that you're already familiar with, please feel free to use it; this book does not require nor assume that you're using 1st Page.

DOWNLOADING AND INSTALLING 1ST PAGE

Before downloading 1st Page, you'll need a program called **WinZip** that allows you to unzip compressed files (i.e., files that end with the .zip extension). It may be the case that you already have WinZip on your computer. To see if this is the case, click on your Windows **Start** button and see if WinZip, for example, appears as one of your programs. If not, you can download an evaluation version for free at the WinZip website. If you have WinZip already, skip ahead to Step 5. Otherwise, begin at Step 1 below to download and install WinZip.

1. Go to the website for WinZip: http://www.winzip.com.

2. Click on the Download Evaluation Version link.

3. Click on link for the recent version of WinZip from the WinZip server. At the time of this writing, the link was labeled Download WinZip 8.1 SR-1. Once you've clicked this link, a File Download window will open. Save the file winzip81.exe to your Desktop. The file should begin downloading automatically.

4. Double-click on the winzip81.exe file on your Desktop in order to install the WinZip program.

5. Go to the website for 1st Page: http://www.evrsoft.com/.

6. Click on the Download Now link.

> **Note.** If the file is not available on the Eversoft web page, there are other places where it can be downloaded. I have up-to-date links to places where 1st Page can be downloaded on the web page for this book: http://www.web-research-design.net.

7. Click on the icon or button that allows you to download the most recent version of 1st Page and follow the instructions.

8. A Download File window will open. Save the file (e.g., 1stpage2.zip) to your Desktop.

9. Right-click on the 1stpage2.zip file on your Desktop. Select the option

Extract to folder C:\Windows\Desktop\1stpage2. This option allows you to use WinZip to unzip the program to a folder called 1stpage2 on your Desktop.

10. Open the 1stpage2 folder on your desktop, and double-click the setup.exe program icon.

11. 1st Page should now be successfully installed.

WHAT IS REQUIRED IN ALL HTML PAGES

Let's create our first web page together. Begin by opening a new document in your text editor. (To do this in 1st Page, click on the File menu, then select the following options: New > Blank Document. A blank page should appear in your 1st Page editor window.)

All HTML pages typically contain the following default commands.

```
<HTML>
<BODY>

</BODY>
</HTML>
```

The things enclosed in the "less than" (<) and "greater than" (>) symbols are called **tags**—programming commands that are used to modify the contents of a web page. All HTML tags are enclosed by "less than" and "greater than" symbols, thereby allowing the browser to distinguish regular text from HTML code. Many, but not all, opening tags require a closing tag, which contains a backslash (e.g., </HTML>). Throughout this book, I will capitalize the commands within tags to help separate them from the rest of the text. It is not necessary that you do this, but you may find it helpful for organizing your code.

The first tag, <HTML>, tells the browser that it is about to receive HTML information. The closing tag, </HTML> tells the browser that the HTML code is complete. The BODY tag isn't necessary unless you want to alter certain page attributes, such as the background color. We'll probably want to change these attributes on occasion, so I've included the BODY tag above.

Go ahead and type these basic tags into your new document. We'll build on these basics in the examples that follow.

> **Note.** Technically, the <HTML> tags are not necessary for most web applications because browsers often assume that they are receiving HTML code. Nonetheless, it is generally considered good form to include these tags in your pages.

CREATING TEXT

To insert some text into your web page, all you have to do is type the text that you would like to appear when someone views your web page. For example, let's say I wanted to create a home page for my study that lists the name of the study and explains its purpose. The following HTML code would do the trick.

example1.htm

```
<HTML>
<BODY>
The purpose of this experiment is to learn more about
    the way we perceive others.
</BODY>
</HTML>
```

This code (1) informs the browser that it is about to receive HTML instructions (line 1), (2) instructs the browser to print the text "the purpose of this experiment is to learn more about the way we perceive others" to the main body of the web page (i.e., the page itself, not the header or title bar) (lines 2 and 3), and (3) informs the browser that is has finished sending body and HTML information (the last two lines). Try typing this into your document, and save the file as **example1.htm**. You'll want to save this file (and all HTML documents we create) to your server's **Public HTML** folder (see Chapter 2 if you don't remember where your **Public HTML** folder is located).

> **Note.** If you are using a professional web hosting service, such as Netfirms, you will need to save the file to your local computer first and then transfer it to the appropriate folder on your server using your FTP program. In this book, when I instruct you to save a file as **example1.htm**, for example, in your **Public HTML** folder, you should (1) save the file as

> **example1.htm** somewhere on your computer, (2) open your FTP program and establish a connection with the server, and (3) transfer the file **example1.htm** on your computer to the **Public HTML** folder on the server. *You will need to follow this general procedure for all the HTML examples discussed in this book.* If you chose to set up your own server instead of using a web hosting service, then I will assume that you are working on your server and you should simply save the file in the appropriate location on your server (i.e., C:\Program Files\Apache Group\Apache2\htdocs\); there will be no need to transfer a file from one location to another.

> **Note.** HTML documents are often saved with the **.htm** or **.html** extension. For the sake of consistency, I will use the .htm extension for the HTML files discussed in this book.

Let's see how the page looks. Open your computer's web browser and type in your site's URL, followed by "example1.htm." For example, the version of **example1.htm** on my server is located at the following web address: http://www.web-research-design.net/example1.htm. You should see something similar to the page depicted in Figure 3.1.

> **Note.** When writing HTML code, it is often useful to have your browser window open. That way you can see what your page looks like as you edit it and save it to the server. To do this, however, you'll need to **Refresh** or **Reload** your page each time you edit it and save it to the server because your browser keeps a copy of the web page stored in memory. Thus, once you've loaded a page, your computer will not continue to reload the contents continually. If the code for the page changes on the server, your browser won't know that unless you explicitly ask it to "reload" the page.

> **Note.** One of the useful features of 1st Page is that it has a preview pane built into it, so you don't necessarily need to open your browser to see what the page will look like. Simply click the **Preview** tab near the top of the window in order to switch between the HTML code and the browser-like interpretation of that code.

PAGE PROPERTIES

You can easily manipulate certain features of your web page, such as the background color and the title of the page (specifically, the title that appears on

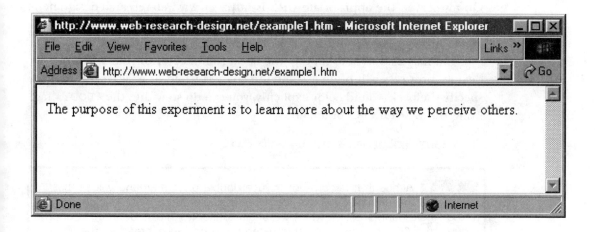

FIGURE 3.1. A basic HTML web page.

the browser's bar). The title of the page is critical because it is the title that many search engines use to index web pages. You should include a title for your page that is as descriptive as possible. Think of the title as an advertisement for your page. If you want people doing web searches on terms such as "personality tests" to find your site, you might want to title your page "Free Psychology Experiments and Personality Tests." If you don't want people to discover your page via a simple web search (e.g., the page represents a specific condition in an experimental design that you don't want people to see unless they are doing the experiment per se), then you should consider omitting the title.

To create a title, use the <TITLE> tag. Here is an example:

example2.htm

```
<HTML>
<TITLE>Social Perception Experiment</TITLE>
<BODY>
The purpose of this experiment is to learn more about
  the way we perceive others.
</BODY>
</HTML>
```

Save this file as **example2.htm** in your server's **Public HTML** folder. To see the page on the Internet, type the appropriate URL into your browser window.

On my server, the appropriate URL is http://www.web-research-design.net/example2.htm. Notice that the title of the experiment now appears in the top of the browser bar, as illustrated in Figure 3.2.

You may also want to modify the background color of your web page. By default, browsers will often assume the color is white or gray. If you want to specify the background color explicitly, you can do so within the <BODY> tag, using the BGCOLOR command:

```
<BODY BGCOLOR = 'blue'>
```

> **Note.** Although it is common to use double quotes around values that are assigned in tags, we will use single quotes. The reason for using single quotes is that when we begin to insert HTML code in our CGI programs, the CGI programs will often reserve the double quotes for specific purposes. If we adopt the convention of using single quotes from the outset, we will not run into problems later.

For many colors, you can simply insert common color names (e.g., 'white,' 'blue,' 'red'), as we did in this example. If you want more control over

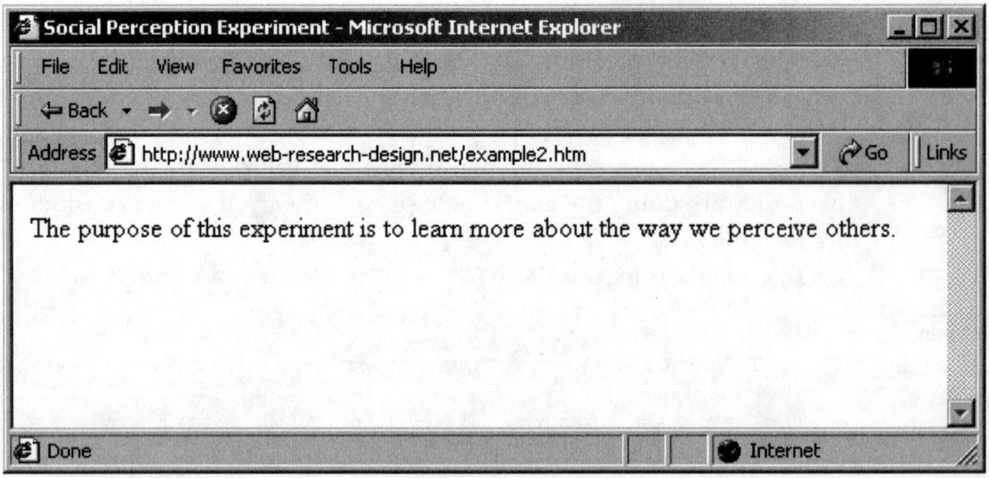

FIGURE 3.2. The title of the page appears in the title bar of the browser window.

the colors you use, you can enter the **hexadecimal** code for various colors. '#ffffff,' for example, is one way of representing white in hexadecimal code. For a thorough discussion of hexadecimal codes and color mixtures, I encourage you to visit the following website: http://www.w3schools.com/html/html_colors.asp.

You may also specify the color of your text in the <BODY> tag using the TEXT command. (The default text color is black on most browsers.)

```
<BODY BGCOLOR = 'blue' TEXT = 'white'>
```

FORMATTING TEXT

At times you will want to modify the appearance of some of your text. For example, you may want to place some words in bold, italicize others, or use different font sizes throughout a document. Here are some commands for some common formatting alternatives. Type these commands between the BODY tags of your document to see how they affect the appearance of text in the browser window. (You may want to enter all of these commands into your document at the same time and then save the file to your server's Public HTML folder and view the results.)

Bold

Use the <B> tag to place your text in boldface.

```
I want the following words <B>to appear in boldface
type</B>, but not these.
```

Italics

Use the <I> tag to italicize text.

```
I would like to <I>italicize</I> some words.
```

Font

To change the font face, use the <FONT> tag with the FACE attribute.

```
Some words look nice in <FONT FACE =
'arial'>arial</FONT>, whereas others look better in
<FONT FACE = 'courier'>courier.</FONT>
```

Text Size

Use the <FONT> tag with the SIZE attribute to alter the size of your text.

```
Some words are <FONT SIZE = '5'>bigger</FONT> than
others.
```

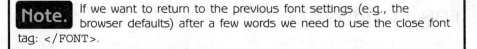 If we want to return to the previous font settings (e.g., the browser defaults) after a few words we need to use the close font tag: </FONT>.

Text Color

If we want to set some text in a different color than the rest of the text (specified in the BODY tag), we can use the <FONT> tag with the COLOR attribute.

```
Some words are <FONT COLOR= 'red'>read</FONT> more
than others.
```

Line Spacing

Even if you type your text on different lines in your text editor, the browser will not display the text on different lines unless you specifically ask it to do so. The tag for a line break is <BR>.

```
I want this to appear on one line. <BR>
And this to appear on the next. <BR>
<BR>
<BR>
This line will be separated from the previous by two
blank lines.
```

Note. There are also paragraph tags (i.e., <P> and </P>) that allow you to separate lines of text into discrete paragraphs. We will not use the paragraph tag much in this book because the same result can be achieved with the <BR> tag.

Centering Text

By default, the text will be "flush left"—aligned against the left-hand side of the page. If you would like to center certain portions of the page, you can use the <CENTER> tag.

```
<CENTER>
Results
</CENTER>
The age and sex breakdown for the sample is presented
    in Table 1.
```

Blank Space

One interesting feature of HTML is that you cannot insert two or more blank spaces into your text unless you specifically request it. Thus, while you can insert a blank space after the end of a sentence by simply using the space bar, you cannot hit the spacebar twice to insert two blank spaces.

To insert more than one character's worth of blank space, you'll need to use a special command: . Here is how it is used:

```
Two blank spaces follow this period.  Nice,
    isn't it?
```

Here is another way to accomplish the same feat, based on the idea that we can get away with creating one space by using the spacebar:

```
Two blank spaces follow this period.  Nice, isn't
    it?
```

Let's combine some of this stuff into a single file and see what it looks like. Copy the following HTML code to a blank document and save it as **example3.htm** in your server's Public HTML directory. View the page in your browser by typing the appropriate URL. (On my server, the URL is http://www.web-research-design.net/example3.htm.)

example3.htm

```
<HTML>
<TITLE>Social Perception Experiment</TITLE>
<BODY BGCOLOR='gray' TEXT='white'>

<B>Social Perception Experiment </B><BR><BR>
```

```
The purpose of this experiment is to learn more about
    the way we perceive others. <BR><BR><BR>
I want the following words <B> to appear in boldface
    type</B>, but not these.<BR>

I would like to <I> italicize</I> some words.<BR>
Some words are <FONT SIZE = '5'> bigger</FONT> than
    others.<BR>
Some words look nice in <FONT FACE = 'arial' COLOR =
    'black'> arial</FONT>, whereas others look better
    in <FONT FACE = 'courier' COLOR = 'black'>
    courier.</FONT>

Two blank spaces follow this period.  Nice,
    isn't it?
</BODY>
</HTML>
```

The web page generated by this code should look similar to that depicted in Figure 3.3.

INSERTING AN IMAGE

To place an image in your document, you'll need to do one of two things. First, if you want to use an image that already exists somewhere on the WWW, you'll need to know the full URL for the image. Alternatively, if you want to place a new image on the Internet (e.g., an image you've scanned or created yourself), you'll need to place that image in your server's Public HTML folder. The URL for the image then becomes the root URL for your site plus the image name. For example, if I wanted to use an image called figure1.jpg, I would save it to my Public HTML folder, and the URL for the image would become http://www.web-research-design.net/figure1.jpg.

For the purposes of keeping your server files organized, I recommend creating a special folder called images in which to store your image files. The tip box explains how to do this, depending on whether you're using a web hosting service or your own server; *the code examples in this book assume that you have a special folder called* images *in your* Public HTML *directory.*

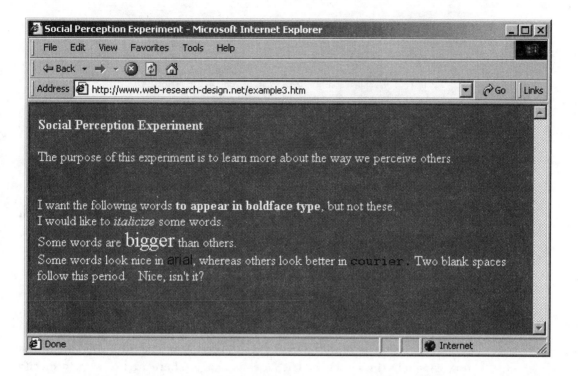

FIGURE 3.3. This web page illustrates the effects of a variety of HTML tags on text appearance.

Tip   Creating a New Image Folder

If you are using Netfirms: Use your FTP program to establish a connection to the server. Open your **www** folder and click the **MkDir** button to create a new directory. Type in, "images" and click **OK**. You should now have a new folder called **images** located *within* your **Public HTML** or **www** directory. You should save any image files you wish to use to this directory.

If you are using your own server: Use your **My Computer** application on the desktop to go to the following location: **C:\Program Files\Apache Group\Apache2\htdocs**. While in your **htdocs** folder, click **File > New > Folder**. Name the new folder "images" by clicking on the name area once and then typing the new name. You should now have a new folder called **images** located within your **Public HTML** or **htdocs** directory. You should save any image files you wish to use to this directory.

Tip   **Saving the Images Used in This Book to Your Server**

To save the images used in this book to your server, go to the web page for this book (http://www.web-research-design.net/) and go to the <u>Downloads</u> section. You will be able to download all of the images used in the book from that site by right-clicking on the image's filename and choosing **Save Target As**, which allows you to save the image to your computer. If you're using your own server, you'll need to save the image to your **images** directory in your **Public HTML** folder. If you're using a professional hosting company, save the image to your computer and then FTP the image to the **images** directory of your **Public HTML** folder.

Once the image has been saved to the **images** folder of your server, you can display the image on your web page by using the <IMG> command. Here is an example:

```
This child can program in Perl.<BR> <BR>
<IMG SRC = '/images/figure1.jpg'>
```

Place this code between <BODY> tags. The web page generated by this code should look similar to that illustrated in Figure 3.4. The SRC attribute of the image tag tells the server the URL for the image. There are two ways to specify this address. First, we can use an "absolute path"—a path that specifies the full

This child can program in Perl.

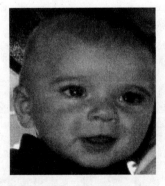

FIGURE 3.4. Using images in a web page.

URL for the image. If we wanted to use an absolute path in the example above, we could set the SRC attribute to "http://www.web-research-design.net/images/figure1.jpg." Second, we can use a "relative path"—a path that expresses the location of the file relative to the current web page. In the example above we have used a relative path. Because the user is already accessing a web page on my site with the base URL http://www.web-research-design.net/, all I need to do is specify the part of the URL that extends the current URL. In this case, all I need to do is specify "/images/figure1.jpg." The server will automatically tack this extension to the URL of the current page (i.e., http://www.web-research-design.net), thereby requesting an image from http://www.web-research-design.net/images/figure1.jpg. I will be using relative paths in this book so that my code will work the same way on your server as it does on mine. In your examples, the relative path "/images/figure1.jpg" will pull the images from the **images** folder on *your* server; in my case, it will pull the images from the **images** folder on *my* server.

If you specify the tag in this way, the image will appear at its *natural* size or dimensions (i.e., the size of the image itself). If you want to adjust the size of the image, you can do so using the size attributes (HEIGHT and WIDTH) of the IMG tag. The metric is pixels, the itty-bitty pieces of light on your screen. Here is an example:

```
Which of the following faces seems more friendly?<BR>
<IMG SRC = '/images/figure1.jpg'>
<IMG SRC = '/images/figure1.jpg' WIDTH = '280' HEIGHT
   = '181'>
```

This code should generate the web page illustrated in Figure 3.5.

It might be useful to specify the width and height attributes when you have visual stimuli that you would like to present in the same dimensions, but the graphics files are not *exactly* same dimensions. As long as the original files are not too different in their dimensions, this method will allow you to present the stimuli in a standard size without distortion.

> **Note.** Remember that, if you alter the HTML code to experiment with these examples, you will need to "refresh" or "reload" the page in your browser in order to see the effect of the changes.

As a general rule, it is better to save the image using the desired dimensions than to adjust the dimensions for which the image is presented. Images

Which of the following faces seems more friendly?

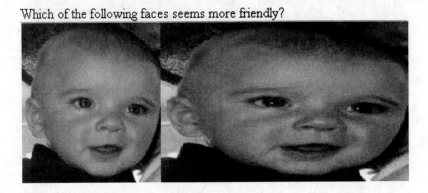

FIGURE 3.5. Adjusting image dimensions on a web page.

can take a while for people to download, so you don't want your users to spend a lot of time downloading large image files that you plan on downsizing in the presentation mode. If you wish to use images in your research but do not already have the images that you would like to use, you should consider obtaining some software that will allow you to create and edit image files. Adobe Photoshop (http://www.adobe.com/products/photoshop/main.html) is a very popular program for image manipulation. The program I use is Paint Shop Pro (http://www.jasc.com/).

CREATING HYPERLINKS

One of the useful features of web pages is the ability to click on a hyperlink in order to instantly jump to another web page. To create a hyperlink, you can use the <A> or anchor tag. Here is an illustration:

```
For more information about this book, please click
   <A HREF = 'http://www.web-research-design.net'>
   here</A>.
```

The URL that you would like to refer your user to when he or she clicks on the link is specified by the HREF attribute. This code should generate a web page that resembles the one depicted in Figure 3.6.

For more information about this book, please check here.

FIGURE 3.6. A hypertext link.

Notice that the text that we wanted to turn into a hyperlink falls between the opening tag and the closing tag. Notice also that the HREF attribute is used to specify the full web address or URL for the link. If the link goes to another file within the same directory as the current page, the full extension will not be necessary and you can use a "relative" link. For example, if I wanted to create a link from **example1.htm** to a file called **example2.htm**, I could use either of the following two HTML commands: <A HREF = 'http://www.web-research-design.net/example2.htm'> Click here to go to the next page </A> or <A HREF = '/example2. htm'> Click here to go to the next page </A>. In either case, when the user clicks on the text that reads Click here to go to the next page, the user will be taken from **example1.htm** to **example2.htm**.

USING IMAGES AS LINKS

There may be times when you find it useful to use an image instead of text as a link. To do this, you insert HTML code for the image, instead of text, in between the hyperlink tags. Here is an example:

```
Please click on the image below for more information
    about the book. <BR>
<A HREF = 'http://www.web-research-design.net'>
<IMG SRC = 'http://www.web-research-design.net/
    images/relationalstructures.jpg'>
</A>
```

This code will produce the web page illustrated in Figure 3.7. Again, absolute or relative paths can be used to specify the URL for the image. If I had used a relative path in this example, I would need to first download the **relationalstructures.jpg** image file to my server's **images** directory.

Please click on the image below for more information about this book.

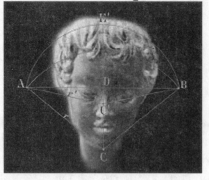

FIGURE 3.7. An image-based link.

USING TABLES EFFECTIVELY

Oftentimes, you'll find it useful to place images, text, or response scales within a table. There are three tags involved in creating a simple table: (1) a <TABLE> tag, used to begin and end the table contexts; (2) a row tag, <TR>, used to begin and end a row; and (3) a column tag, <TD>, used to begin and end the contents of a column within a row. Here is an example:

```
<TABLE>
<TR>
<TD>
first row, first column
</TD>
<TD>
first row, second column
</TD>
</TR>
<TR>
<TD>
second row, first column
</TD>
<TD>
second row, second column
</TD>
</TR>
</TABLE>
```

Notice that the flow of commands is row by column. In other words, we first begin a row using <TR>, then create the columns *within that row* using <TD> and </TD>, then we end the row with </TR> and begin again with the next row. The web page generated by this code is illustrated in Figure 3.8. Notice that, by default, the columns are as wide as the contents of the largest cell. It is noteworthy that we didn't need to tell the browser how many rows or columns we were going to use; we simply used as many as we needed. This feature will turn out to be very convenient later when we discuss ways to customize experimental feedback for subjects but don't know in advance how many rows will be necessary.

It is not necessary that each command be placed on a separate line. (In fact, an entire HTML file could be written on a single line, if desired!) Here is the way I would typically format the previous set of commands in my text editor:

```
<TABLE>
<TR>
<TD>first row, first column</TD>
<TD>first row, second column</TD>
</TR>
<TR>
<TD>second row, first column</TD>
<TD>second row, second column</TD>
</TR>
</TABLE>
```

The <TABLE> tag has a number of attributes that allow you to alter the appearance of the table in ways that may be useful. For example, you can create a border for the table by adding the BORDER attribute to the <TABLE> tag. Also, you can alter the color of the border using the BORDERCOLOR attribute. You can adjust the spacing between cells and the padding between cells by adding the CELLSPACING and CELLPADDING attributes to the <TABLE> tag. The CELLSPACING tag affects the amount of pixel space between different cells in the table. If this attribute is set to 2, then a 2-pixel

first row, first column   first row, second column

second row, first column second row, second column

FIGURE 3.8. A basic table.

space will be placed between all the cells in the table. The CELLPADDING tag affects the amount of pixel space between the borders of the cell and the contents of the cell. If this attribute is set to 5, a 5-pixel space will be placed between the edges of the cell and the contents of the cell. Here is an example of how some of these attributes affect the appearance of a table. I encourage you to experiment with different pixel sizes so you can see how these attributes affect the appearance of the table.

```
<TABLE BORDER CELLSPACING = 2>
<TR>
<TD>first row, first column</TD>
<TD>first row, second column</TD>
</TR>
<TR>
<TD>second row, first column</TD>
<TD>second row, second column</TD>
</TR>
</TABLE>
```

This code will produce the table illustrated in Figure 3.9.

There will be situations in which you want a particular row of the table to span one or more columns. You can span both columns and rows by using the COLSPAN and ROWSPAN attributes within a <TD> or <TR> tag, respectively. Here is an example.

```
<TABLE BORDER CELLSPACING = 2>
<TR>
<TD COLSPAN='2'>Factor A</TD>
</TR>
<TR>
<TD>Level 1</TD>
<TD>Level 2</TD>
</TR>
<TR>
```

first row, first column	first row, second column
second row, first column	second row, second column

FIGURE 3.9. A table with borders.

```
<TD>4.50</TD>
<TD>2.46</TD>
</TR>
<TR>
<TD>8.7</TD>
<TD>5.6</TD>
</TR>
</TABLE>
```

In this code, we have set COLSPAN to 2, thereby instructing the browser to create a row that spans or crosses 2 columns. The table created by this code is illustrated in Figure 3.10. For more information on the various ways you can create and format tables, please visit the following link: http://www. w3schools.com/html/html_tables.asp. We will be using some of the tricks described on that page later in this book, such as aligning and centering elements within columns or rows.

> **Note.** Unfortunately, the various text attributes you define in an HTML document (e.g., font face, font color) do not apply to the cells within a table. If you don't want to use the browser defaults for elements within a table, you'll need to retype these attributes within each cell of a table. I will illustrate how to do this in the next example.

BRINGING IT ALL TOGETHER

Okay, now let's use these basic tools to create a home page for your website. The purpose of this page will be to introduce visitors to the kinds of research you're conducting. Although we haven't created any online research studies

Factor A	
Level 1	Level 2
4.50	2.46
8.7	5.6

FIGURE 3.10. A table in which one row spans two columns.

yet, I'll create links to some of my online studies for the purpose of illustration. You may want to copy this code and modify the contents to convey information about the kinds of research you plan to conduct online.

In this example, we'll illustrate the use of the TABLE tag to format text. We'll also use links and images, as well as different kinds of fonts and text sizes. You may or may not want all these tweaks on your own site, but I want to show you how these commands work.

home.htm

```
<HTML>
<TITLE> Online Attachment Style Survey </TITLE>
<BODY>

<TABLE>
<TR>
<TD BGCOLOR = '333366'>
<IMG SRC = '/images/relationalstructures.jpg'>
</TD>

<TD><FONT FACE = 'Times' SIZE = '5'>Online Attachment
   Style Surveys </FONT><BR><BR></TD>
</TR>

<TR>
<TD BGCOLOR = '333366'></TD>
<TD>
<FONT FACE = 'arial' SIZE = '2'>
The objective of this site is to provide up-to-date
   links to interactive web surveys on adult
   attachment styles. Each of these interactive
   questionnaires takes less than 10 minutes to
   complete, and will provide you with immediate
   feedback on aspects of your interpersonal style.
<BR><BR><BR>

<A HREF = 'http://P034.psch.uic.edu/crq.htm'><B>Adult
   Attachment Style</B></A><BR><BR>
People differ considerably in how secure or insecure
   they feel in their close relationships. This 7-minute
   interactive questionnaire is designed to assess how
   secure or insecure you feel in your close
   relationships. When you are finished answering the
   questions, the program will tell you about your
   attachment style.
<BR><BR><BR>
<A HREF = 'http://p034.psch.uic.edu/Claudia/relstructures.
   htm'><B>Relational Structures </B></A><BR><BR>
```

```
We do not always relate in the same way to different
    people in our lives. We might feel insecure with
    our parents, for example, but secure in our current
    dating or marital relationships. This 10-minute
    interactive questionnaire will ask you some
    questions about the way you relate to five
    important people in your life, and provide you with
    feedback on the structure of your mental
    representations of those relationships.
</FONT>
<BR><BR><BR><BR>

<FONT FACE = 'arial' SIZE = '1'>
For questions about this website, please contact Chris
    Fraley at fraley@uic.edu.</FONT>
</TD>
</TR>
</TABLE>

</BODY>
</HTML>
```

Copy this code to a blank document in your text editor, modify it accordingly, and save it as home.htm in your Public HTML directory. Next, enter the URL for the page in the address bar of your web browser. On my server, the appropriate URL is http://www.web-research-design.net/home.htm. The web page generated by this code is illustrated in Figure 3.11.

> **Note.** To view a web page, you will almost always need to type the name of the web page (e.g., home.htm) in addition to the URL of the website. However, as you will notice if you go to the website for this book (i.e., http://www.web-research-design.net/), you will see a web page without having typed in the name of a specific page. Although the name of the file was not listed in the URL, the file does have a name: index.htm. Files with the name index.htm or index.html are often displayed *automatically* by web servers when a user specifies only a directory and not a specific file. If you would like your home.htm page to be the default page that is displayed when a user enters in the root of your URL, you'll need to do two things. First, you'll need to delete or rename all the files in your Public HTML directory that have "index" as their name. Second, you'll need to rename your home.htm file is index.htm or index.html. After doing this, you should see your new page by default when you enter the root URL (e.g., http://www.web-research-design.net/) in the browser address bar.

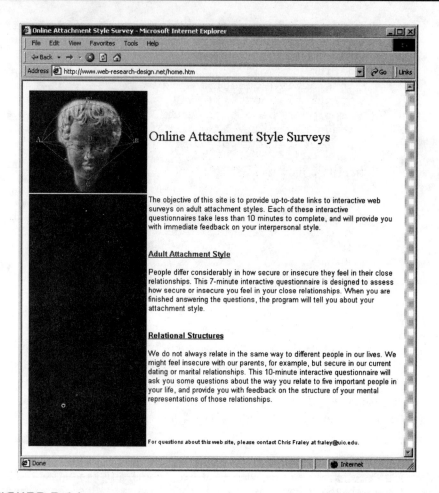

FIGURE 3.11. An example web page that combines many of the HTML commands we have discussed.

SUMMARY

In this chapter you have learned how to make a basic web page. Let's review some of the key points:

1. HTML "tags" are used to convey instructions to the browser about how to display information.

2. All web pages should begin with a <HTML> tag and close with a </HTML> tag.

3. Many, but not all, starting tags require an ending or closing tag. For example, when you want to place some text in bold, you need to surround the appropriate text with a <B> tag to instruct the browser to begin using bold typeface and a </B> tag to instruct the browser to stop using bold typeface.

4. You can use HTML tags to affect the appearance of text, including the font, the font size, font color, and centering.

5. To include a line break, use the <BR> command. The <BR> command does not require a "closing" or "end" tag.

6. To instruct the browser to display an image, use the <IMG> tag. In this tag, you must specify the URL for the image's location using the SRC or "source" attribute. You can specify the URL using an absolute path (e.g., <IMG SRC = 'http://www.web-research-design.net/images/figure1.jpg'>) or a relative path (e.g., <IMG SRC = '/images/figure1.jpg'>). You can also adjust the width and height of the displayed image using the WIDTH and HEIGHT attributes.

7. You can create a link to another web page by using the <A> tag. Use the HREF attribute to specify the URL for the web page to which you'd like to link. For example, the HTML tag <A HREF = 'http://www.guilford.com'>Click here to go to the Guilford Press website</A> will create a hyperlink to the Guilford Press website.

8. Tables are a useful tool for organizing the placement of text and images. To begin and end a table, use the <TABLE> and </TABLE> tags, respectively. To create a new row, use the <TR> tag. To create a new cell within a row, use the <TD> tag to begin the cell and the </TD> tag to end the cell. Use the </TR> tag to end a row.

9. Basic HTML pages should be saved to the Public HTML directory on your server. If you're using the Netfirms web hosting service, your Public HTML directory is labeled "www." If you've created your own Apache server, your Public HTML directory is labeled "htdocs."

In the next chapter, we'll explore HTML *forms*—ways of obtaining input or responses from the person using the page.

Here is a review of some basic HTML codes. Many of these were discussed in this chapter; some of them will be discussed in subsequent chapters but are included here for easy reference.

HTML tag	Function	Example

`<HTML>`
`</HTML>`
	Instructs the browser that the document contains HTML code. This tag should be placed at the beginning of each HTML document you create, and a corresponding `</HTML>` tag should be placed at the end.	`<HTML>`
		`contents of web page`
		`</HTML>`

`<BODY>`
`</BODY>`
	The body tag is used to specify the properties (e.g., background color) of an HTML document.	`<BODY BGCOLOR = 'blue'>`
		`contents of web page`
		`</BODY>`

`<B>` `</B>`	Instructs the browser to place the text in bold type.	This `<B>`word`</B>` will appear in bold type.
`<I>` `</I>`	Instructs the browser to place the text between the tags in italics.	`<I>`This sentence will be italicized.`</I>`
`<FONT>` `</FONT>`	Sets the properties of the font (e.g., the color, size, and type face).	`<FONT SIZE = '2' COLOR= 'gray' TYPE= 'arial'>` `text appears here </FONT>`
` `	Creates a line break. (No closing tag is required.)	Line 1 ` ` Line 2
`<CENTER>` `</CENTER>`	Centers the text and images between tags.	`<CENTER>General Discussion</CENTER>`
` `	Instructs the browser to include a blank space within the text. Without this command, you can only place one space between words.	Extra ` ` ` ` spaces

`<IMG>`	Inserts an image into an HTML document. The SRC or source attribute is used to specify the URL (using a relative or absolute path) for the image file to be displayed. Additional attributes, such as WIDTH and HEIGHT can be used to adjust the dimensions (in pixels) of the image.	Using an absolute path to the image:
		`<IMG SRC = 'http://www.web-research-design.net/images/figure1.jpg' WIDTH = '280' HEIGHT = '171'>`
		
		Using a relative path to the image:
		`<IMG SRC = '/images/figure1.jpg' WIDTH = '280' HEIGHT = '171'>`

`<A>`
`</A>`
	Creates a hyperlink. The HREF attribute specifies the URL (using a relative or absolute path) for the linking page. Text or images can be transformed into links by placing them between the opening and closing tags.	Using an absolute URL:
		`<A HREF = 'http://www.web-research-design.net/page2.htm'> Click here to link to go to Page 2</A>`
		
		Using a relative URL:
		`<A HREF = '/page2.htm'> Click here to link to go to Page 2 </A>`

HTML tag	Function	Example

`<TABLE>` `</TABLE>`	Instructs the browser to create a table. The table tag has several optional attributes that can be specified. The BGCOLOR attribute sets the background color of the table. The BORDER attribute specifies, in pixels, how thick the borders of the table should be. The BORDERCOLOR attribute specifies the color of the border. The BACKGROUND attribute places an image in the background of the table. The CELLSPACING and CELLPADDING attributes specify, in pixels, how much space to place between cells and how much space to place between the border of a cell and its contents, respectively.	`<TABLE BGCOLOR= 'red' BORDER = '1'>table contents</TABLE>`
		
		 or
		
		 `<TABLE BACKGROUND = '/images/figure1.jpg' CELLPADDING = '2'>table contents</TABLE>`

`<TR>` `</TR>`	Instructs the browser to construct a new row within a table. The `<TR>` tag must be enclosed within the `<TABLE>` open and close tags. The closing tag is used to denote the end of the row: `</TR>`.	`<TABLE>` `<TR>` this is the first row in my table `</TR>` `<TR>` this is the second row in my table `</TR>` `</TABLE>`
`<TD>` `</TD>`	Instructs the browser to construct a new cell within a row of the table. The `<TD>` tag (and its close tag, `</TD>`) must be nested within a table row. Optional attributes: The WIDTH attribute specifies, as a percentage, the proportion of the table that should be devoted to the width of the cell. The WIDTH attribute only needs to be specified in one row. The VALIGN attribute aligns the cell contents vertically with the top, center, or bottom of the cell. The ROWSPAN and COLSPAN attributes allow the cell to span a specified number of rows or columns, respectively.	`<TABLE>` `<TR>` `<TD WIDTH = '80%' VALIGN = 'top'> cell 1</TD>` `<TD WIDTH = '20%' VALIGN = 'top'> cell 2 </TD>` `</TR>` `<TR>` `<TD VALIGN = 'bottom'> cell 3 </TD>` `<TD VALIGN = 'bottom'> cell 4 </TD>` `</TR>` `</TABLE>`

Chapter 4

HTML Forms

Collecting Research Data from Participants via the Internet

You have probably seen web pages on the Internet that ask the user to enter information. For example, you may have been asked to enter your mailing address on an online order form, or to use a rating scale to rate your satisfaction with a product. These "input" abilities are made possible by the use of *forms*. **Forms** are special areas of a web page that allow the user to provide information (e.g., written comments, ratings, selections from menus) that is processed by the server.

There are four main components to a form.

- First, there is the **form tag**, which tells the browser that this part of the HTML page will be used to gather information. A form begins with the <FORM> tag and ends with the </FORM> tag.
- Second, there are **attributes** within the <FORM> tag that tell the browser what to do with the input once the **Submit** button (see below) has been pressed. For the purposes of this book we'll cover two options: (1) the data will be e-mailed to a specified e-mail address (the researcher's) or (2) the

data will be sent to a CGI script on the server that will process the data (e.g., manipulate it or save it to a data file).

Third, there is a way for the **user to provide data**. The user may provide data by means of typing, checking checkboxes, clicking a button, or selecting from a list in a pull-down menu.

Fourth, there is a **Submit** button that the user will click when he or she is finished with his or her responses. Sometimes these buttons say "submit," or something else, such as "go to checkout." Image links can also be used as **Submit** buttons.

Let's discuss each of these of these components in turn. Then, we'll walk though a couple of examples to help illustrate the use of forms in simple data collection.

THE FORM TAG

To create an area of the web page that will accept input from the user, you'll need to use the <FORM> tag. Here is an example of such a tag:

```
<FORM ACTION = 'mailto:fraley@uic.edu' METHOD = 'post'
   ENCTYPE = 'text/plain'>
```

There are three key attributes in this tag. The first, ACTION, tells the browser what to do when the user clicks the **Submit** button. We will be dealing with two kinds of actions: (1) actions that involve sending the data to the researcher via e-mail and (2) actions that involve sending the data to the server for CGI processing. For the purposes of this chapter, however, we will only deal with the e-mail option. *You'll need to substitute your e-mail address for mine in the code above.*

> **Note.** Form data can only be submitted via e-mail if the user's computer is configured correctly. If you're using your office or lab computer to check e-mail on a regular basis, then your computer probably is configured correctly for you to do these demonstrations, although your computer may "warn" you that you are about to submit data over the Internet. As a general rule, you will not want to collect data via e-mail in a real research context

> because participants may be using computers (e.g., computers in public labs) that are not configured for e-mail. In addition, the use of e-mail will reveal the participant's user name, which may compromise the confidentiality of the data. In the next chapter I'll show you how to have the data sent from a form to the server without using e-mail.

The second key attribute is the METHOD attribute. For virtually everything we'll be doing, this will be set to *post*.

The third attribute, ENCTYPE, is used only when we are sending the data via e-mail. This instructs the browser to send the data as simple, unencrypted text. (You should not send the data encrypted unless you have special software for decrypting the data. Moreover, without encryption, you should not request private or personal data from your participants.)

CREATING RESPONSE WINDOWS AND RATING SCALES

There are many ways to use forms to collect responses from the user. We will discuss many highly versatile and simple techniques here, including text boxes, radio buttons, pull-down menus, checkboxes, and coordinate maps. In this section I'll outline the basics of these different techniques for collecting information. Once I've introduced each of these techniques, we'll work through a handful of examples so that you can see exactly how the different components (e.g., the <FORM> tags, the **Submit** button) are configured on a web page.

Text Boxes

A text box is a region on the screen in which a user can type (or paste) a response. The text box option is highly useful if you're collecting narrative data, or if you want users to be able to give you comments that are not constrained by rating scales.

Here is the HTML code for creating a simple text box; the output of this code is illustrated in Figure 4.1.

```
<INPUT TYPE = 'text box' NAME = 'v1' MAXLENGTH = '25'
   SIZE = '25'>
Please enter your codename or alias.<BR>
```

`spappy|`   Please enter your codename or alias.

FIGURE 4.1. A text box is one way to collect text-based information from users.

Please note the MAXLENGTH and SIZE attributes of this tag. The SIZE attribute determines how large the text box area will be on the screen. The MAXLENGTH attribute determines how many characters (e.g., letters) will be permitted in the box. If you need to collect a lot of information, it is wise to set this attribute to a high value. If you do not need to collect a lot of typed information, however, set it to a small value. If this value is not constrained in some manner, troublemakers may paste pages and pages of text into these boxes in an attempt to overwhelm or crash your server.

It is okay to set the SIZE attribute smaller than the MAXLENGTH attribute. The browser will store all the typed information, even if the entire text cannot be viewed at once.

Here is another way of creating a text box called TEXTAREA; the web page generated by this code is illustrated in Figure 4.2.

```
Please tell us what you think about this
   experiment.<BR>
<TEXTAREA NAME = 'v1' COLS = '20' ROWS = '6' WRAP =
   'virtual'>
Please type here.
</TEXTAREA>
```

Please tell us what you think about this experiment.

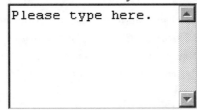

FIGURE 4.2. A text area box provides a way to collect multiple lines of text from a user.

The <TEXTAREA> tag, like the <INPUT> text box tag, allows the user to input text. However, this tag is a bit more flexible and allows you to specify the rows (ROWS) and columns (COLS) of the input area as attributes. In addition, the NAME attribute is used to name the input and the WRAP attribute can be set to 'virtual' (which allows the text to wrap around the box) or 'off' (which does not force the text to wrap). The <TEXTAREA> tag requires a close tag: </TEXTAREA>. You can place precreated text within the opening and closing tags, and this text will automatically appear when the HTML page is loaded.

> **Tip**   A neat feature of the TEXTAREA option is that you can place pretyped text within the box. Thus, if you were doing an experiment on education or learning that required people to proofread and correct a text, you could place the stimulus text within the box, instruct participants to correct it, and then you would receive the revised text as the response.

In both the <INPUT> text box and the <TEXTAREA> tags, we had an attribute called NAME. This attribute provides a name for the response (e.g., a variable label or name). When the data are e-mailed to you (or later sent to a CGI script), the response to this input box will be prefaced by the variable name. For reasons that will be explained in subsequent chapters, I will adopt the convention of appending "v", for variable, and a number for my major variable names (e.g., v12 will be variable 12). When there will be more than 10 variables, I will use v01, v02, v03, and so on instead of v1, v2, v3, for the first 9 variables.

Radio Buttons

Radio buttons are a remarkably flexible tool for collecting data. They are most useful when several response options exist for a question, and you don't want the user to be able to select more than one option per question. Here is some example HTML code for two radio buttons:

```
Are you Female or Male?<BR>
<INPUT TYPE = 'radio' NAME = 'v2' VALUE = 'F'> Female
   <BR>
```

```
<INPUT TYPE = 'radio' NAME = 'v2' VALUE = 'M'> Male
   <BR>
```

The appearance of this code on a web page is illustrated in Figure 4.3.

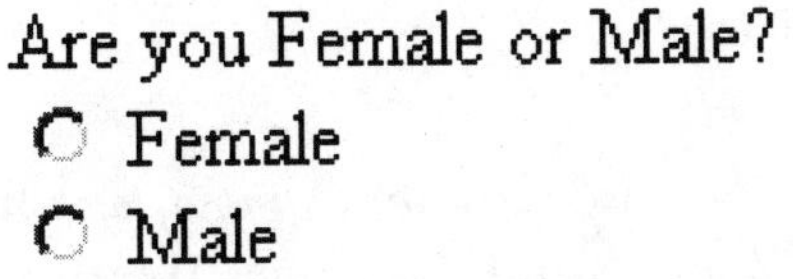

Are you Female or Male?
    ○ Female
    ○ Male

FIGURE 4.3. Radio buttons can be used to collect responses to mutually exclusive options.

There are two important things to note here. First, for each response option (male and female), there is a separate <INPUT> tag. Notice, also, that these tags do not need to be closed (i.e., there is no backslash tag). Second, in this example, the options are construed as being mutually exclusive. If someone selects "Female" and then selects "Male," the previous selection of "Female" will disappear. In short, we've created two radio buttons, each with the same name (v2). v2 can only have one value, so when one option is selected, the other cannot be. It is important to note that we did *not* use the same variable name that we have used for previous questions (e.g., the text box example).

Multiple radio buttons can be strung together to create a rating scale. Here is an example of how this can be achieved:

```
I believe that American corporations have too much
   power.<BR>
Strongly Disagree
<INPUT TYPE = 'radio' NAME = 'v3' VALUE = '1'>
<INPUT TYPE = 'radio' NAME = 'v3' VALUE = '2'>
<INPUT TYPE = 'radio' NAME = 'v3' VALUE = '3'>
<INPUT TYPE = 'radio' NAME = 'v3' VALUE = '4'>
<INPUT TYPE = 'radio' NAME = 'v3' VALUE = '5'>
<INPUT TYPE = 'radio' NAME = 'v3' VALUE = '6'>
<INPUT TYPE = 'radio' NAME = 'v3' VALUE = '7'>
Strongly Agree
<BR>
```

The output of this code is illustrated in Figure 4.4.

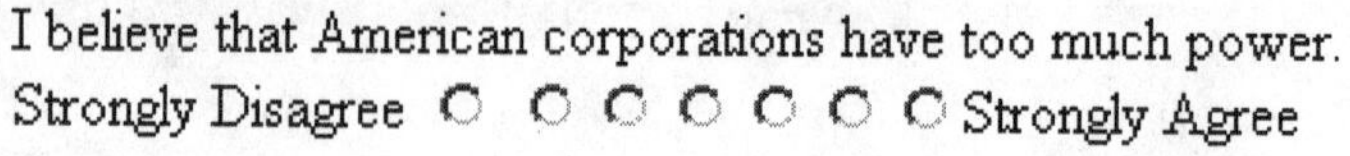

I believe that American corporations have too much power.
Strongly Disagree ○ ○ ○ ○ ○ ○ ○ Strongly Agree

FIGURE 4.4. The use of radio buttons to obtain scaled ratings.

Notice that we used a *separate input tag* for each radio button, but used the *same name* (i.e., v3) for each one. We also assigned a different numeric value to each radio button to quantify the person's rating. If the user clicks the right-most radio button (i.e., the one next to the "Strongly Agree" label), the value of v3 will be set equal to 7; if the user clicks the left-most radio button, the value of v3 will be set to 1.

> **Tip**   It is possible to have one radio button in a set preselected in order to create a "default" response. For example, if we wanted the mid-point of the scale to be pre-selected, we would alter the corresponding INPUT tag from the previous example as follows: `<INPUT TYPE = 'radio' NAME = 'v3' VALUE = '4' CHECKED>`. When the web page is displayed for the user, the fourth response option will already be selected. The user will have to choose another response option if he or she believes the default option is inappropriate.

> **Note.**   It is important to keep in mind that, if you have several radio buttons as response options for a single stimulus or questionnaire item, the NAME attribute needs to be the same for all of the radio buttons. When there are two or more radio buttons with the same NAME attribute, the user can only select one of those buttons. This is true even if the buttons are not in close proximity to one another on the web page. If you have a radio button named "v03" at the top of the page and another one named "v03" at the bottom of the page, the user can only select one of these buttons. Please make sure that all of your buttons for a single stimulus have the same name and that you use a different name for different stimuli.

Pull-Down Menus

Pull-down menus are useful when you have a large (but not too large) number of response options and you would like your user to select one. I often use these menus when subjects are indicating their sex, ethnicity, or country of origin. Caution: Pull-down menus eat up a lot of memory on your user's browser. If you use more than twenty of these menus, the page may become distorted.

```
I am the kind of person who likes to program.
<SELECT NAME = 'v4' SIZE = '1'>
<OPTION VALUE = '0' SELECTED>---Please select an
    option---</OPTION>
<OPTION VALUE = '1'>Strongly Disagree</OPTION>
<OPTION VALUE = '2'>Disagree</OPTION>
<OPTION VALUE = '3'>Agree</OPTION>
<OPTION VALUE = '4'>Strongly Agree</OPTION>
</SELECT>
```

Figure 4.5 illustrates the way this code would be translated by a browser.

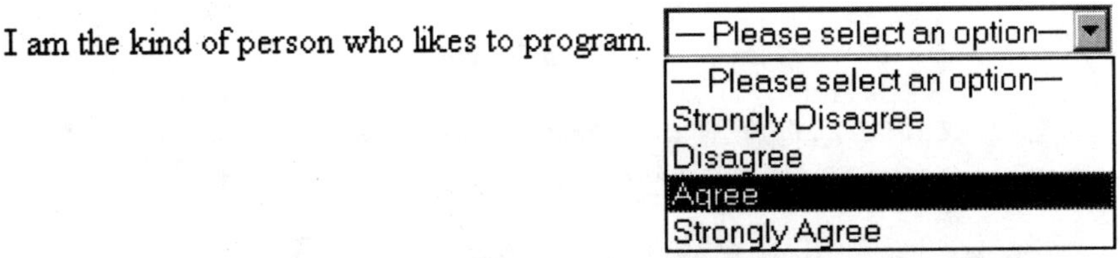

FIGURE 4.5. A pull-down menu can be used to display several response options when the user clicks on the menu.

Notice that there are several tags required to create a pull-down menu. The first pair of tags, `<SELECT>` and `</SELECT>`, instructs the browser to create a pull-down menu and, in this example, label the user's response under the variable NAME v4. The SIZE attribute is used to indicate how many options are viewable prior to opening the menu. The second pair of tags, `<OPTION>` and `</OPTION>`, is used to create each menu option. Notice that separate option tags are required for each menu option that exists. The VALUE attribute of the option tag is used to specify the value (quantitative or qualitative) assigned to a specific selection. Also notice that I added the attribute SELECTED to the first menu option. This attribute instructs the browser to preselect the first option. If the user does not select another option, the variable v4 will automatically be coded as a "0" in this example—a value that represents a nonresponse. Both the SELECT and OPTION tags require closing tags.

Checkboxes

Checkboxes can be useful when you have a list of options that you want the user to check, if applicable. For example, if you have a list of affective states (e.g., sad, happy, bitter), you may ask a user to check each affective state that describes the way he or she feels at the moment.

```
Please check the adjectives that describe your mood
    right now. <BR>
<INPUT TYPE ='checkbox' NAME ='v01' VALUE ='1'> Sad
    <BR>
<INPUT TYPE ='checkbox' NAME ='v02' VALUE ='1'> Happy
    <BR>
<INPUT TYPE ='checkbox' NAME ='v03' VALUE ='1'>
    Anxious <BR>
<INPUT TYPE ='checkbox' NAME ='v04' VALUE ='1'> Sleepy
    <BR>
```

Figure 4.6 illustrates the way the checkboxes will appear in the browser window. (I've taken the liberty of checking the "happy" and "sleepy" boxes in Figure 4.6.) Notice that the user can select as many or as few items as he or she likes. In order to accomplish this, however, each checkbox needs a separate name. It is helpful to think about each checkbox option as representing a separate item, and that the user can respond to it or not.

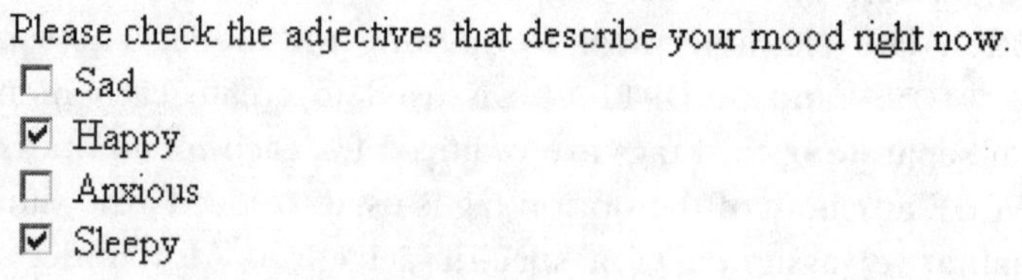

Please check the adjectives that describe your mood right now.
- ☐ Sad
- ☑ Happy
- ☐ Anxious
- ☑ Sleepy

FIGURE 4.6. Checkboxes can be used when the response options are not mutually exclusive.

THE SUBMIT BUTTON

Once the user is finished responding to all the questions or stimuli, he or she will need to click on a special button to tell the browser that he or she has finished filling in the form. Once the button is pressed, the data are either sent to a specified e-mail address or are processed by a CGI script. (Which of these two things happens will depend on the way the METHOD attribute was specified in the FORM tag.) Here is the HTML code for creating a submit button.

```
<INPUT TYPE = 'submit' VALUE = 'Please click here
   when finished'>
```

Figure 4.7 shows how this code will appear on a web page, combined with the select menu discussed previously. The VALUE attribute contains the text that will be placed inside the button—the button label. By default, the text will read "Submit" or "Submit Query," but you may want to make it more informative, such as "Click here to continue."

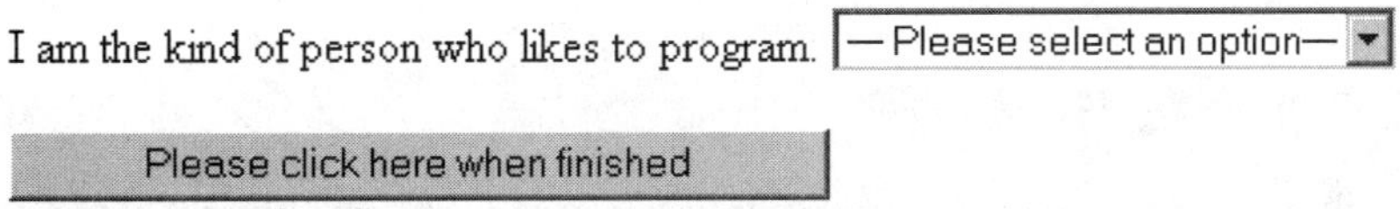

I am the kind of person who likes to program. | — Please select an option— ▼ |

| Please click here when finished |

FIGURE 4.7. A **Submit** button.

IMAGE MAPS

Image maps can be used to collect data from participants in many creative ways. An image map tag instructs the browser to present an image to the user. When the user clicks on the image, the browser submits the x (horizontal) and y (vertical) coordinates for the specific pixel location in the image clicked by the user. (The coordinate 0, 0 denotes the top-left corner of the image). Thus, the image acts as a **Submit** button while also serving as a way to collect information.

To see how an image map works, consider the following example. We've asked the user to rate his or her mood on a continuous scale. The scale itself, however, is an image rather than a series of radio buttons. All the user needs to do is click somewhere along the scale, and the precise location of the click (i.e., the *x* and *y* coordinates) will be recorded as the user's response.

```
How are you feeling right now?<BR><BR>
Please click anywhere on the scale below to indicate
   your current mood. <BR>
<BR><INPUT TYPE='image' SRC='/images/imagemap1.jpg'
   NAME='coord'>
```

Figure 4.8 provides an illustration of the way a browser may render this code. When the user clicks somewhere along this scale, both the *x* and *y* coordinates of the click will be recorded and the data will be submitted. Because there are two pieces of information associated with the click (the coordinates corresponding to the *x* and *y* axes), the browser will append "x" and "y" to the NAME attribute of the image map when submitting the data. In this example, the value corresponding to the *x* axis would automatically be labeled "coord.x" by the browser and the value corresponding to the *y* axis would automatically be labeled "coord.y." We'll discuss image maps again in Chapter 9.

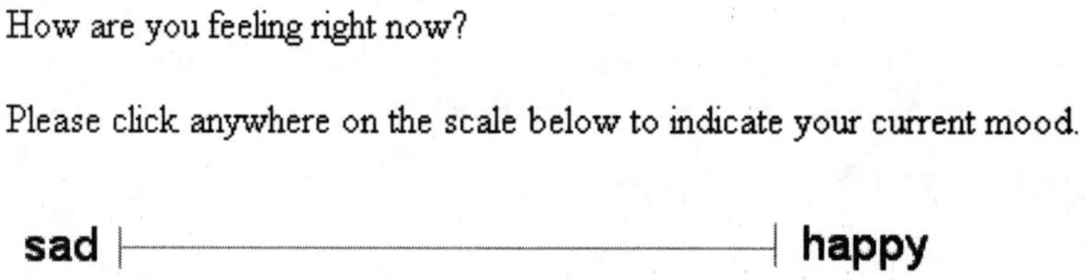

How are you feeling right now?

Please click anywhere on the scale below to indicate your current mood.

sad |—————————————————————| **happy**

FIGURE 4.8. The use of an image map as a way to both collect ratings and to submit the data.

HIDDEN TAGS

Sounds secretive, right? Hidden tags are tags that you place in a form that contain useful information, but not information that the user will see. The concept is best illustrated by example.

```
<INPUT TYPE = 'hidden' NAME = 'v0' VALUE =
  'MoodSurvey'>
```

When the submit button is clicked, I will be e-mailed the user's responses, as well as the contents of the hidden tag. In this case, the value of this variable, which is called v0, is the name of the survey. If I have multiple surveys online at once, this piece of information will let me know which survey the data have come from. As will be illustrated in the examples below, the user will not be able to see this variable on the actual web page; it is hidden from view.

> **Note.** Hidden tags are absolutely essential for designing complex Internet experiments. There may be cases in which we want to collect data from the user via multiple web pages (e.g., each page contains a stimulus from a different level in a within-subjects manipulation). Hidden tags can be used to store the user's responses to each stimulus so we can carry that information forward from one page to the next. These tags may seem mysterious and even pointless right now, but their power will become more apparent in subsequent chapters.

TWO EXAMPLES

Let's illustrate everything we've discussed thus far with a simple example. In this example, we will create a page that asks the participant four simple questions. This will allow us to explore several of the input techniques we have discussed up to this point: radio buttons, pull-down menus, text boxes, and checkboxes. When the user is finished, he or she can click on a **Submit** button, and the data will be e-mailed to the researcher. Copy this code to a blank document and save it as **examplesurvey1.htm** in your Public HTML directory. (You'll need to change the e-mail address from mine to yours.) Feel free to edit it and experiment with it. To view the file in your browser window, enter the appropriate URL for the page in your browser address bar. On my server, the URL is http://www.web-research-design.net/examplesurvey1.htm.

examplesurvey1.htm
```
<HTML>
<FORM ACTION = 'mailto:fraley@uic.edu' METHOD = 'post'
  ENCTYPE = 'text/plain'>
```

```
<INPUT TYPE = 'hidden' NAME = 'v0' VALUE =
   'ExampleSurvey'>Welcome to our survey! <BR><BR>
1. Which of the following foods do you enjoy? (Check
   all that apply) <BR>
<INPUT TYPE = 'checkbox' NAME = 'v1' VALUE = '1'>
   Spinach <BR>
<INPUT TYPE = 'checkbox' NAME = 'v2' VALUE = '1'>
   Eggplant <BR>
<INPUT TYPE = 'checkbox' NAME = 'v3' VALUE = '1'>
   Rice <BR>
<INPUT TYPE = 'checkbox' NAME = 'v4' VALUE = '1'>
   Anything deep fried <BR><BR><BR>

2. My country of origin is: <BR><SELECT NAME = 'v5'
   SIZE = '1'>
<OPTION VALUE = '0' SELECTED>---Please select an
   option---</OPTION>
<OPTION VALUE = '1'>USA</OPTION>
<OPTION VALUE = '2'>CANADA</OPTION>
<OPTION VALUE = '3'>MEXICO</OPTION>
<OPTION VALUE = '4'>OTHER</OPTION>
</SELECT><BR><BR>

3. I believe that corporations have too much power.
<BR>Strongly Disagree
<INPUT TYPE = 'radio' NAME = 'v6' value='1'>
<INPUT TYPE = 'radio' NAME = 'v6' value='2'>
<INPUT TYPE = 'radio' NAME = 'v6' value='3'>
<INPUT TYPE = 'radio' NAME = 'v6' value='4'>
<INPUT TYPE = 'radio' NAME = 'v6' value='5'>
<INPUT TYPE = 'radio' NAME = 'v6' value='6'>
<INPUT TYPE = 'radio' NAME = 'v6' value='7'>
Strongly Agree<BR><BR>

4. Please tell me what you think of this book so
   far.<BR>
<TEXTAREA NAME = 'v7' COLS = '20' ROWS = '6' WRAP =
   'virtual'>Please type here.</TEXTAREA><BR>

<INPUT TYPE = 'submit' VALUE = 'Please click here
   when finished'>
<BR><BR>Thank you for your participation!
</FORM></HTML>
```

Figure 4.9 illustrates the web page generated by this code.

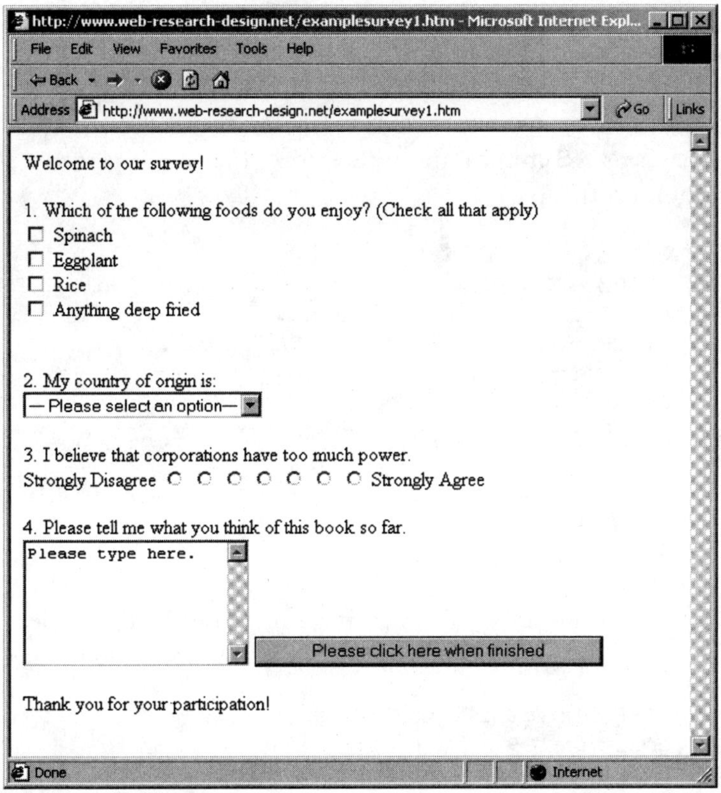

FIGURE 4.9. This web page illustrates many of the different response options that we have discussed.

Finally, here is what the contents of the e-mail might look like:

```
v0=ExampleSurvey
v2=1
v4=1
v5=1
v6=6
v7=I like this book so far, Chris. I think it will
    be very helpful as I design my online studies.
```

Notice that information about v1 and v3 were not sent via e-mail because those options were not selected. As a general rule, the browser will only e-mail responses to questions, not nonresponses. In Chapter 5 we will discuss ways of recording nonresponses to questions.

Here is another example that involves the use of an image map. (I have saved it as ex--samplesurvey2.htm on my server.) Recall that an image map behaves as a **Submit** button; therefore, I have not placed a separate **Submit** button on this page.

examplesurvey2.htm

```
<HTML>
<FORM ACTION = 'mailto:fraley@uic.edu' METHOD = 'post'
    ENCTYPE = 'text/plain'>
<INPUT TYPE = 'hidden' NAME = 'v0' VALUE =
    'ExampleSurvey2'>Welcome to our survey! <BR><BR>
Please rate your current mood on the scale below.
    Please click somewhere on the scale to indicate how
    sad or happy you are feeling.<BR><BR>
<INPUT TYPE='image' SRC='/images/imagemap1.jpg'
    NAME='coord'>
</FORM></HTML>
```

Figure 4.10 illustrates the web page rendered by this code.

Here is what the contents of the e-mail might look like:

```
v0=ExampleSurvey2
coord.x=199
coord.y=25
```

In this particular example, the y-coordinate doesn't mean too much. We may, however, take the x-coordinate as a continuous measure of a user's current mood.

Here is one more example. I am not introducing any new tricks here, but I will incorporate some of the formatting codes from the previous chapter in order to illustrate some ways to make a simple questionnaire look more professional. Specifically, I will use the TABLE tag to help format and align some of the questions, and I'll include an image to make things look nicer. Copy this code to a blank document, modify the e-mail address, and save it as moodsurvey.htm in your Public HTML folder.

moodsurvey.htm

```
<HTML>
<TITLE> Mood Questionnaire | HTML Demonstration
    </TITLE>
```

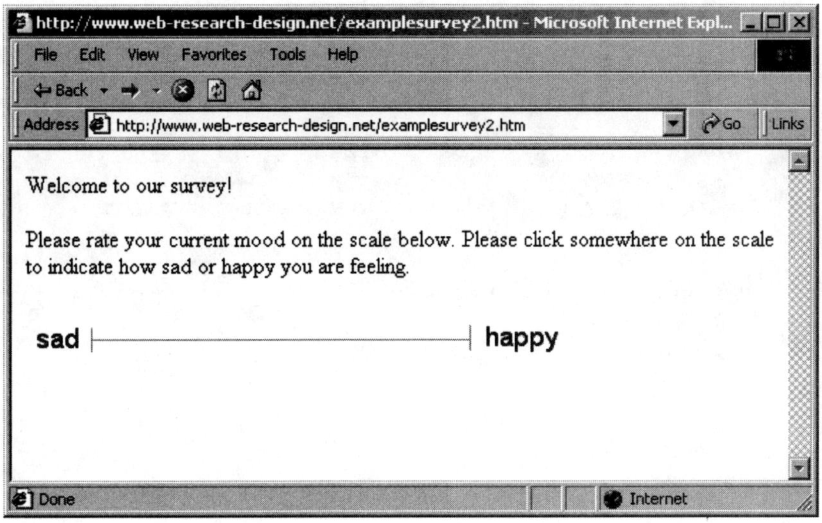

FIGURE 4.10. An image map to collect and submit data.

```
<FORM ACTION = 'mailto:fraley@uic.edu' METHOD = 'post'
  ENCTYPE = 'text/plain'>
<INPUT TYPE = 'hidden' NAME = 'v0' VALUE =
  'MoodSurvey'>

<TABLE CELLPADING = '2'>

<TR>
<TD bgcolor = '000066'><IMG SRC =
  '/images/relationalstructures.jpg'></TD>
<TD><FONT FACE = 'arial' SIZE = '5'> Mood
  Questionnaire </TD>
</TR>

<TR>
<TD bgcolor = '000066'></TD>
<TD>
<FONT FACE = 'arial' SIZE = '2'>
Please indicate whether you are <I>currently</I>
  experiencing the following mood states.<BR><BR>

<TABLE>
```

```
<TR>
<TD>
<FONT FACE = 'arial' SIZE = '2'>
<B>happy </B>     </TD>
<TD>
<FONT FACE = 'arial' SIZE = '2'>
<I>no</I>
<INPUT TYPE = 'radio' NAME = 'v1' VALUE = '0'>
</TD>
<TD>
<INPUT TYPE = 'radio' NAME = 'v1' VALUE = '1'>
<FONT FACE = 'arial' SIZE = '2'>
<I>yes</I>
</TD>
</TR>

<TR>
<TD>
<FONT FACE = 'arial' SIZE = '2'>
<B>anxious</B>     </TD>
<TD>
<FONT FACE = 'arial' SIZE = '2'>
<I>no</I>
<INPUT TYPE = 'radio' NAME = 'v2' VALUE = '0'>
</TD>
<TD>
<INPUT TYPE = 'radio' NAME = 'v2' VALUE = '1'>
<FONT FACE = 'arial' SIZE = '2'>
<I>yes</I>
</TD>
</TR>

<TR>
<TD>
<FONT FACE = 'arial' SIZE = '2'><B>curious</B>  
     </TD>
<TD>
<FONT FACE = 'arial' SIZE = '2'>
<I>no</I>
<INPUT TYPE = 'radio' NAME = 'v3' VALUE = '0'>
</TD>
<TD>
<FONT FACE = 'arial' SIZE = 2>
<INPUT TYPE = 'radio' NAME = 'v3' VALUE = '1'>
<I>yes</I>
```

```
</TD>
</TR>
<TR>
<TD>
<FONT FACE = 'arial' SIZE = '2'><B>sorrowful </B> 
     </TD>
<TD>
<FONT FACE = 'arial' SIZE = '2'>
<I>no</I>
<INPUT TYPE = 'radio' NAME = 'v4' VALUE = '0'>
</TD>
<TD>
<INPUT TYPE = 'radio' NAME = 'v4' value='1'>
<FONT FACE = 'arial' SIZE = '2'>
<I>yes</I>
</TD>
</TR>
</TABLE>

<BR><BR>
<FONT FACE = 'arial' SIZE = '2'>
<INPUT TYPE = 'submit' VALUE = 'Click here when
   finished'>
<BR><BR>
<I>Thank you for your participation!</I>
</FORM>

</TD>
</TR>

</TABLE>
</HTML>
```

Figure 4.11 illustrates the way the file should look in your browser (on my server, the appropriate URL is http://www.web-research-design.net/ moodsurvey.htm). When the user clicks the **Submit** button, an e-mail will be sent to my account that contains each variable (e.g., v1, v2) and the corresponding response (coded as 0 for "no" and 1 for "yes"):

```
v0=MoodSurvey
v1=1
v2=0
v3=1
v4=0
```

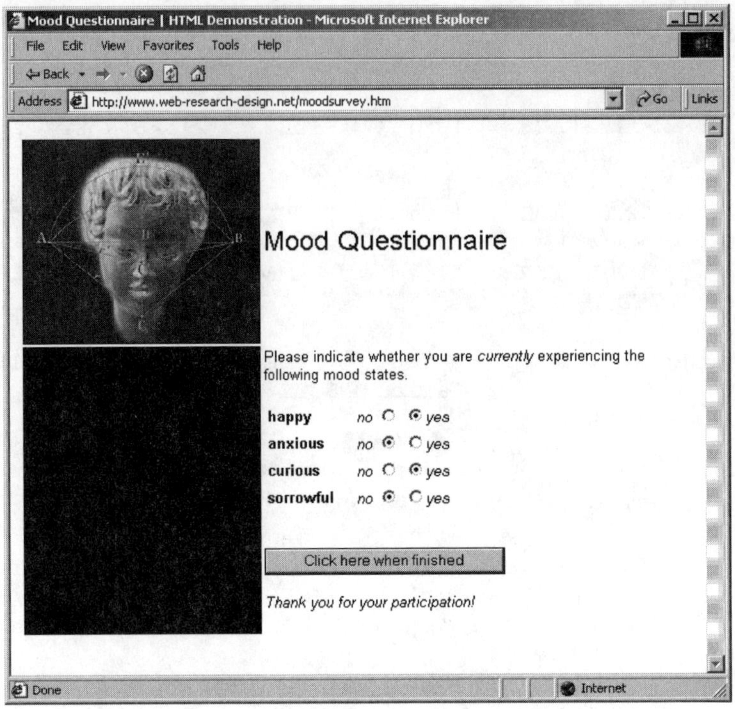

FIGURE 4.11. This page combines some of the form elements we have discussed, along with some of the formatting commands reviewed in Chapter 3.

Note. You may be wondering why we didn't use checkboxes in this example. In this example, the two options, "yes" and "no," are mutually exclusive responses to the items. If we use radio buttons, we can assign the "yes" and "no" responses for any one item to have the same name. This ensures that one selected option will disappear if the other is selected. With checkboxes, this is not the case. Even if multiple checkboxes are given the same name, checking one will not "uncheck" the others. If we had used checkboxes in this example, we would have asked the user only to check the box if the answer was "yes"; there would have been no box to choose for a "no" response.

One of the advantages of conducting research over the Internet is that you can program your server to automatically store the data. It isn't such a bad thing to receive data via e-mail if you're polling a handful of people on an issue. If you have hundreds of people participating in your research, however, you don't want to have your mailbox cluttered with hundreds of e-mails. In the next chapter, I'll show you how to have the data automatically stored as a text file (one that can be imported easily into Microsoft Excel or SPSS) on your server. This will provide us with an excellent transition into programming in Perl, and using CGI scripting to your advantage.

Here is a review of the HTML codes that pertain to input forms. Many of these were discussed in this chapter; but, in some cases I have included additional attributes that were not discussed that you may find useful.

HTML tag	Function	Example
`<FORM>` `</FORM>`	Creates an "input" area in which the user can provide information. The `<FORM>` tag has several attributes. The ACTION attribute tells the browser what to do when the submit button is pressed. This attribute specifies an e-mail address or the URL for a CGI script that will process the data. The METHOD attribute indicates the manner in which the form data will be sent. (In this book, we will always set this attribute to "post.") When the data are being sent by e-mail, specify the ENCTYPE or encryption attribute. (In this book we will always set this attribute to "text/plain.")	To send data to an e-mail address: `<FORM ACTION = 'mailto: fraley@uic.edu METHOD = 'post' ENCTYPE = 'text/plain'>` Input area and **Submit** button `</FORM>` To send data to a CGI script: `<FORM ACTION = '/cgi-bin/scriptname.pl' METHOD = 'post'>` input area and **Submit** button `</FORM>`
`<INPUT TYPE = 'textbox'>`	The text box is a method of input that allows the user to type his or her responses. This tag has several attributes. The NAME attribute specifies the name of the variable that corresponds to the input. The MAXLENGTH attribute specifies the number of characters that can be entered. The SIZE attribute specifies the number of characters that can be viewed at once inside the box.	Please type your comments here. `<INPUT TYPE = 'textbox' NAME = 'comments' MAXLENGTH = '200' SIZE = '50'>`
`<TEXTAREA>` `</TEXTAREA>`	The `<TEXTAREA>` tag allows the user to input text. It also allows you to specify the rows (ROWS) and columns (COLS) of the input area. The NAME attribute names the input. The WRAP attribute should be set to "virtual" (which allows the text to wrap around the box) or "off" (which does not force the text to wrap). You can place precreated text between the opening and closing tags.	`<TEXTAREA NAME = 'mylife' COLS = '20' ROWS = '20' WRAP = 'virtual'> Please tell us a bit about your life here. </TEXTAREA>`

(cont.)

HTML tag	Function	Example
`<INPUT TYPE = 'radio'>`	This tag creates a single radio button that the user can click. Radio buttons are often used to create rating scales in which each button corresponds to a different rating but where only one rating is permitted. The NAME attribute names the input information. The VALUE attribute assigns a quantitative or qualitative value to the variable when the button is pressed. If the CHECKED attribute is specified, the button will automatically be selected and the user will have to deselect it.	`Are you a coffee fan? ` `No <INPUT TYPE = 'radio'` `NAME = 'variable1' VALUE =` `'no'> ` `Yes <INPUT TYPE = 'radio'` `NAME = 'variable1' VALUE =` `'yes'>` or `Are you a coffee fan? ` `No <INPUT TYPE = 'radio'` `NAME = 'variable1' VALUE =` `'1' CHECKED> ` `Yes <INPUT TYPE = 'radio'` `NAME = 'variable1' VALUE =` `'2'>`

`<SELECT>`
`</SELECT>`
and
`<OPTION>`
`</OPTION>`
	The `<SELECT>` tag allows users to use a pull-down menu to make their selections. The NAME attribute names the input. The SIZE attribute indicates how many options are viewable prior to opening the menu. Each option is specified using the OPTION tag. The VALUE attribute specifies the value (quantitative or qualitative) assigned to a specific selection. Both the `<SELECT>` and `<OPTION>` tags require close tags. The SELECTED attribute can be specified within an option if you would like it to be preselected.	What is your coffee preference?
		
		`<SELECT NAME = 'coffee'`
		`SIZE = '1'>`
		`<OPTION VALUE = '1'>no`
		`coffee</OPTION>`
		`<OPTION VALUE = '2'`
		`SELECTED>black</OPTION>`
		`<OPTION VALUE = '3'>with`
		`cream</OPTION>`
		`<OPTION VALUE = '4'>black`
		`with sugar</OPTION>`
		`<OPTION VALUE = '5'>cream`
		`and sugar please</OPTION>`
		`</SELECT>`

`<INPUT TYPE = 'submit'>`	Creates a **Submit** button. This button must be pressed by the user in order for the form information to be sent to the researcher. The VALUE attribute specifies the text that will appear on the button itself. This tag does not require a close tag.	`<INPUT TYPE = 'submit'`
		`VALUE = 'press this button`
		`to go to the next page'>`

`<INPUT TYPE = 'image'>`	The image `<INPUT>` tag creates an image map input area. When a user clicks on the image, the form information is automatically submitted, along with the x and y coordinates (in pixels) of the clicked location in the image. The SRC (or source) attribute specifies the URL for the image to be used as a map. The NAME attribute names the x and y coordinates that are submitted. (The browser will automatically append an ".x" and ".y" to the name to distinguish the x and y coordinates.)	`<INPUT TYPE = 'image' SRC`
		`= '/images/imagemap1.jpg'`
		`NAME = 'coord'>`

HTML tag	Function	Example
`<INPUT TYPE = 'hidden'>`	A hidden tag is used to pass along information to the researcher—information that will not appear on the web page itself; it is hidden from the user. The NAME attribute specifies the variable name for the information. The VALUE tag specifies the hidden information to be passed along.	`<INPUT TYPE = 'hidden' NAME = 'condition' VALUE = '2x3'>`
`<INPUT TYPE='password'>`	The password tag creates a textbox in which the user can enter a password. As the user enters the password, the text will be replaced by a series of asterisks. This prevents onlookers from viewing the password. Like a standard text box, the password box has a NAME attribute, a MAXLENGTH attribute, and a SIZE attribute.	`<INPUT TYPE='password' NAME='secretcode' MAXLENGTH='30' SIZE='25'>`

Chapter 5

An Introduction to CGI Scripting

Using Perl to Automatically Save Response Data to a File

Up to now, what we've done has not required server-side programming. In principle, you can use the HTML skills taught in Chapters 3 and 4 to create web pages, collect data, and have the data e-mailed directly to you. However, in order to use the Internet for more sophisticated research purposes, you'll need to have control over how the data are stored, how pages are delivered to the user, and how the stimuli are presented. To accomplish this, you'll need to write programs that run on your server. These programs, or CGI scripts, will give you the power you need to use the Internet in a truly interactive and dynamic way.

As discussed in Chapter 1, CGI stands for common gateway interface—a standard for exchanging information between computers (e.g., the user's computer and the server). We'll be writing our CGI scripts in Perl—a highly flexible programming language, and one that is widely used for CGI programming. We'll begin by discussing a simple script that can be used to take data submitted from an HTML form and save it to a text file database on the server. We won't go into the nuts and bolts of all the programming code; we'll simply use this as an example to introduce you to the process of CGI scripting. In later chapters you'll learn more about how the specific commands operate.

Let's begin by looking at the simple online mood survey from the last chapter (moodsurvey.htm). As you'll recall, the purpose of this survey was to assess whether or not the user was experiencing each of four moods. The original web page was designed to e-mail us the data when the **Submit** button was clicked. Now, however, we want the data to be sent to a program on our server for processing. We can make this change by altering the ACTION attribute of the <FORM> tag. Let's change the form tag from

```
<FORM ACTION = 'mailto:fraley@uic.edu' METHOD = 'post'
    ENCTYPE = 'text/plain'>
```

to

```
<FORM ACTION = '/cgi-bin/savedata1.pl' METHOD =
    'post'>.
```

The complete HTML code for the web page is below. After making the change to the <FORM> tag, save your revised file as moodsurvey2.htm in your **Public HTML** directory.

moodsurvey2.htm

```
<HTML>
<TITLE> Mood Questionnaire | HTML Demonstration
    </TITLE>
<FORM ACTION = '/cgi-bin/savedata1.pl' METHOD =
    'post'>

<INPUT TYPE = 'hidden' NAME = 'v0' VALUE =
    'MoodSurvey'>

<TABLE CELLPADING = '2'>

<TR>
<TD bgcolor = '000066'><IMG SRC =
    '/images/relationalstructures.jpg'></TD>
```

```
<TD><FONT FACE = 'arial' SIZE = '5'> Mood
   Questionnaire </TD>
</TR>

<TR>
<TD bgcolor = '000066'></TD>
<TD>
<FONT FACE = 'arial' SIZE = '2'>
Please indicate whether you are <I>currently</I>
   experiencing the following mood states.<BR><BR>

<TABLE>

<TR>
<TD>
<FONT FACE = 'arial' SIZE = '2'>
<B>happy </B>     </TD>
<TD>
<FONT FACE = 'arial' SIZE = '2'>
<I>no</I>
<INPUT TYPE = 'radio' NAME = 'v1' VALUE = '0'>
</TD>
<TD>
<INPUT TYPE = 'radio' NAME = 'v1' VALUE = '1'>
<FONT FACE = 'arial' SIZE = '2'>
<I>yes</I>
</TD>
</TR>

<TR>
<TD>
<FONT FACE = 'arial' SIZE = '2'>
<B>anxious</B>     </TD>
<TD>
<FONT FACE = 'arial' SIZE = '2'>
<I>no</I>
<INPUT TYPE = 'radio' NAME = 'v2' VALUE = '0'>
</TD>
<TD>
<INPUT TYPE = 'radio' NAME = 'v2' VALUE = '1'>
<FONT FACE = 'arial' SIZE = '2'>
<I>yes</I>
</TD>
</TR>
```

```
<TR>
<TD>
<FONT FACE = 'arial' SIZE = '2'><B>curious</B>  
     </TD>
<TD>
<FONT FACE = 'arial' SIZE = '2'>
<I>no</I>
<INPUT TYPE = 'radio' NAME = 'v3' VALUE = '0'>
</TD>
<TD>
<FONT FACE = 'arial' SIZE = 2>
<INPUT TYPE = 'radio' NAME = 'v3' VALUE = '1'>
<I>yes</I>
</TD>
</TR>

<TR>
<TD>
<FONT FACE = 'arial' SIZE = '2'><B>sorrowful </B> 
     </TD>
<TD>
<FONT FACE = 'arial' SIZE = '2'>
<I>no</I>
<INPUT TYPE = 'radio' NAME = 'v4' VALUE = '0'>
</TD>
<TD>
<INPUT TYPE = 'radio' NAME = 'v4' value='1'>
<FONT FACE = 'arial' SIZE = '2'>
<I>yes</I>
</TD>
</TR>
</TABLE>

<BR><BR>
<FONT FACE = 'arial' SIZE = '2'>
<INPUT TYPE = 'submit' VALUE = 'Click here when
   finished'>
<BR><BR>
<I>Thank you for your participation!</I>
</FORM>
</TD>
</TR>
</TABLE>
</HTML>
```

With this minor change, we are now instructing the user's browser to send the data to a CGI script called **savedata1.pl** located in the **cgi-bin** directory on our server. (Note: If you're viewing **moodsurvey2.htm** on your server, don't click the **Submit** button yet. Before the server can process the data, we need to get **savedata1.pl** up and running.)

> | **Note.** | The **.pl** extension indicates that our script is a Perl program. All of the CGI programs that we write in this book will be written in Perl and will end in the .pl extension. |

SAVING THE DATA VIA A SIMPLE CGI SCRIPT

Now we need to create a program called **savedata1.pl** that will process the data packet that has been sent to our server. We will want this program to do three things. First, we want it to take the data packet being sent by the participant and parse it in a useful way. Second, we want the program to store the relevant data in a text file that can be imported into a popular data-analysis program, such as SPSS, Microsoft Excel, or S-Plus. Third, we want the program to give the user a "thank you" message for his or her participation.

CGI programs, like HTML pages, can be written in a text editor, such as 1st Page. Let's begin, then, by opening a blank document in our text editor. Type the following code into the document, and save the file as **savedata1.pl** in the **cgi-bin** directory of your server. Recall that the **cgi-bin** directory is a different directory from the **Public HTML** directory we were using previously. (Please see Chapter 2 if you can't recall where the **cgi-bin** directory is located.)

savedata1.pl

```
#!C:/perl/bin/perl.exe
use CGI;
$query = new CGI;

$v0= $query->param('v0');
$v1= $query->param('v1');
$v2= $query->param('v2');
$v3= $query->param('v3');
$v4= $query->param('v4');
```

```
open(INFO,
    ">>$ENV{'DOCUMENT_ROOT'}/www/data/moodexample.txt");
print INFO "$v0, $v1, $v2, $v3, $v4 \n";
close (INFO);

print $query->header;
print $query->start_html(-title=>'Thank You');
print "<FONT FACE = 'arial' SIZE = '2'>Thank you for
    your participation in this research! </FONT>";
print $query->end_html;
```

If you're new to CGI programming in Perl, this will probably look a bit over-whelming at first. Don't worry; we're going to break down each step of this program in order to make the operations clear.

The First Line of All Perl Scripts

Here is the first line of the CGI program:

```
#!C:/perl/bin/perl.exe
```

This line tells the server to execute the script using Perl. *This line will need to be the first line in any CGI program you write.* This line, sometimes called the "shebang!" line, directs the server to the Perl program, which should be located at C:/perl/bin/perl.exe. If you've set up your own Apache server, you should double-check this location by searching your computer for the perl.exe file and determining whether it is located in this place. If it is not, then you should adjust the shebang! line so that it specifies the correct path. If you're using a web hosting service, the company's help pages will indicate what to place in the shebang! line. (The line above works on both my Netfirms server and on my Apache server, which I installed using all the default options.)

Instructing the Server to Process the Submitted Data

The next two lines,

```
use CGI;
$query = new CGI;
```

will also be in every CGI script that we discuss in this book. The first of these tells the server to use the common gateway interface to accept the data packet submitted by the user's computer. The data packet will contain a lot of information, including the hidden value that we included in one of the HTML tags (named "v0"), the responses to the four mood items (named "v1," "v2," "v3," and "v4"), and a number of "environment" variables. **Environment variables** include information such as the server's IP address, the URL of the web page that activated or "called" the script, and the user's IP address. We'll discuss some of these environment variables in more detail later. For now, the important thing to know is that the data packet contains a lot of information, only some of which we care about. The next line assigns all of the information in the data packet to the catchall variable "$query."

> **Note.** Each Perl line ends with a semicolon. This is how Perl parses different lines of code. Each distinct line of commands in Perl needs to end with a semicolon.

Extracting Values from the Submitted Data and Assigning Them Variable Names within the CGI Script

The next set of commands demonstrates a very basic function in Perl. In short, these commands allow us to create five new variables (e.g., $v0–$v4) that will be assigned the values contained in $query. The first line, for example, translates to, "Create a new variable called $v0 and let it equal the value of the parameter called 'v0' from $query." Now, there is a Perl variable called $v0. Similarly, the second line says, "Create a new variable called $v1 and let it equal the value of the parameter called 'v1' from $query."

```
$v0= $query->param('v0');
$v1= $query->param('v1');
$v2= $query->param('v2');
$v3= $query->param('v3');
$v4= $query->param('v4');
```

> **Note.** The meaning of the term **variable** in Perl is actually similar to its meaning in standard behavioral research. It refers to something

that can take on one of two or more alternative values. In Perl, all variables are prefaced by the dollar sign. Thus, any time you create or refer to a variable in Perl (e.g., v01), you need to preface it with a dollar sign (e.g., $query). This is how Perl keeps variable names separate from other kinds of objects and commands.

Technically, this kind of variable is a **scalar** variable because it represents a single value. Later, we will discuss variables called **arrays** or **vectors** which contain more than one scalar and are prefaced with an @ symbol (e.g., @v01) instead of a dollar sign. If this terminology seems a bit abstract, here is another way to conceptualize the difference between these two kinds of variables. If we had a scores for five people on an intelligence test, any one person's score would be a scalar variable and would be denoted with a dollar sign (e.g., $IQ). The set of scores for the five people would be an array of intelligence test scores, and would be denoted with an @ (e.g., @IQ). This array, or vector, contains five scalars.

This code creates five new variables to correspond to the pieces of information submitted from the web user (including the information hidden in the "v0" tag). These variables only exist for internal use by the script; this kind of variable is often called a **local variable**.

Writing to a Data File

Now we want to save the values of our new variables to a data file. To do so, we first need to open (or create) a data file, place the values in the file, and then close it.

Here is how it is done in this example program:

```
open(INFO,
    ">>$ENV{'DOCUMENT_ROOT'}/www/data/moodexample.txt");
print INFO "$v0, $v1, $v2, $v3, $v4 \n";
close (INFO);
```

The first line instructs the server to open a file called moodexample.txt in the data folder within your server's Public HTML directory. If the file already exists, then the use of the >> in the path name instructs the server to **append**, or put any new information at the end of, an already existing file. (In other words, we won't copy over any data that are already in the file; we'll simply add more.) If the file does not exist, Perl will create it for us. INFO is called a

file handle, and is a short-cut way to reference the contents of the file within your Perl program. The `$ENV{'DOCUMENT_ROOT'}/www/data/moodexample.txt` part of the code tells the server to locate the moodexample.txt data file in the **data** directory on your server. You'll be storing your data files in the same place (i.e., the "data" directory on your server) for all the examples in this book, so this line (except for the file name at the end) will be the same in all of our examples.

Now that the data file has been opened, we can add new data to it. To do so, we use the **print** command. The print command listed above translates to "Take the values of the variables $v0, $v1, $v2, $v3, and $v4 and place them into the file we've opened."

Notice that we have been separating each of these variables with a comma. The print command takes these commas literally. In other words, the command is printing the values of each of these variables *separated by commas* to the data file. This will allow us to eventually open the file in Microsoft Excel or SPSS as a "comma-delimited" text file, which makes it easy to import data into these programs. If we left the comma out, the values would not be separated from each other, unless we inserted some other symbol, such as a tab or semicolon.

Notice that the last thing we print on that line in the Perl file is \n. This is Perl-speak for a line break, and means that the computer will know to enter any further pieces of data on a new line, or row, in the data file. Without \n, the server would keep appending new data from new subjects at the end of the same line.

Because behavioral scientists generally organize their data spreadsheets in a person-by-variable manner (i.e., persons represent rows and variables represent columns), it is always a good idea to include the \n symbol after the last variable has been entered for a subject. Doing so ensures that the next person who submits data will have their data stored on a new line in the file.

On the next line, the *close* command instructs the server to close (and implicitly, save) the data file. After writing to a data file, you should always close it.

Note. If several people might be simultaneously using a CGI script that writes to a data file, it is possible that the data will be written incorrectly. One solution to this problem is to lock the data file (i.e., prevent others from using it) while a user is running a script that is accessing it. To do this, you can use the **flock** command. Here is an example:

```
open(INFO,
">>$ENV{'DOCUMENT_ROOT'}/www/data/moodexample.txt");
flock(INFO, 2);
print INFO "$v0, $v1, $v2, $v3, $v4 \n";
close (INFO);
```

The flock command doesn't work on all systems. For example, it doesn't work on my Apache server running on Windows 98. It does work, however, on my Netfirms server. You may need to try your program with and without a flock command in order to see whether it will work on your server.

Fortunately, it is unlikely that you will have two people simultaneously writing to a file. The writing process is rather quick and it is unlikely that you will have multiple research participants submitting their data at exactly the same time.

Inserting HTML Code into the CGI Script

The final set of commands allow us to send HTML code to the user's browser. Any time you want to use CGI to create HTML code, the following commands must be included in your script. The first two lines act like the <HTML> tag,

```
print $query->header;
print $query->start_html(-title=>'Thank You');
```

and the last line acts like the </HTML> tag:

```
print $query->end_html;
```

Notice that we can use HTML code in Perl in exactly the same way as we did when working with HTML documents! The only difference is that we now insert the HTML code within double quotations, preceded by a print statement.

```
print "<FONT FACE = 'arial' SIZE = '2'>Thank you for
    your participation in this research! </FONT>";
```

out CGI scripting in Perl is
HTML code we've dis-
ed content to our users
th an extraordinary
ages. For example, as
ithin a CGI script with
itself "create" the web

ay to interweave HTML
ein that is commonly
ll be a few cases in
ables), but as a gen-
I have chosen to do
ML and Perl; to the
so. For more infor-
tein.cshl.org/

TESTING THE CODE

Let's experiment a bit with this program to see exactly how it works. Open the mood questionnaire in your browser and answer the mood questions. (On my server, the appropriate URL is http://webbook.netfirms.com/moodsurvey2.htm.) When you click the **Submit** button, you should see a new web page that says nothing more than, "Thank you for your participation in this research!"

Let's see if the program saved the data successfully. To view your data files, you will need to use one of two methods, depending on whether you are using a web hosting service such as Netfirms or you are using your own Apache server.

• If you are using a web hosting service, establish an FTP connection to your server. Open the data folder within the Public HTML directory. Click once on the data file (e.g., moodexample.txt) to highlight it and then click the green arrow in WS_FTP Pro pointing from the Remote window to the Local window. This will instruct the FTP program to transfer a copy of your data file from the server to your local computer. By default, your FTP program will probably try to save the file to an FTP directory on your computer (e.g., C:\Program Files\WS_FTP\). You may find it easier to transfer the file to another directory, such as your Desktop or a folder that you've created especially for your Internet programs. To select another directory, simply move backwards or forwards through your local directory window.

• If you are using an Apache server, go to the data folder within the www folder of your Public HTML directory. The moodexample.txt data file should be in there.

Using your text editor, open the file called moodexample.txt. You should see something like the following:

```
MoodSurvey,1,0,1,0
```

These values represent the values of the five variables we saved to the datafile: $v0$, $v1$, $v2$, $v3$, and $v4$. These variables were extracted from the responses to the mood questions that the user sent us.

Close the moodexample.txt file and try entering some additional responses using the web page. (In other words, pretend that you're another subject.) Now, open the moodexample.txt file again and see how the program saved the data. (If you're using a web hosting service, don't forget to FTP the data file to your computer again. Once you've submitted additional data, the moodexample.txt file on the server will change, and you'll want to obtain the most recent copy.)

```
MoodSurvey,1,0,1,0
MoodSurvey,0,1,0,1
```

Notice that the new submission is entered as the next line in the data file. Also, notice that the previous submission was not erased.

Before we continue, let's take a moment to see what we've managed to accomplish thus far.

• We've created a web page that uses an HTML form to obtain mood ratings from subjects.

• Once the subject finishes answering the questions and clicks the **Submit** button, his or her responses are sent to the server.

• We've created a simple CGI script called savedata1.pl that is executed when the user submits his or her data.

• The script does three things. First, it extracts the responses (and hidden values) from the submitted data and gives them easy-to-use names (e.g.,

$v1) within the script itself. Second, it opens (or creates, if need be) a data file called moodexample.txt and saves the user's data as a new line in that file. Third, it sends HTML code back to the user to thank him or her for participating.

The script we just created is a very useful one for saving our mood data. Moreover, it can be easily modified to save data from other kinds of web studies. For example, let's assume we had created 11 questions, and, in the HTML code, the responses to each set of radio buttons were named "v00" to "v10." In order to read these values in from the data packet, we could expand the first section of our CGI script to

```
$v00= $query->param('v00');
$v01= $query->param('v01');
$v02= $query->param('v02');
$v03= $query->param('v03');
$v04= $query->param('v04');
$v05= $query->param('v05');
$v06= $query->param('v06');
$v07= $query->param('v07');
$v08= $query->param('v08');
$v09= $query->param('v09');
$v10= $query->param('v10');
```

and

```
open(INFO,
    ">>$ENV{'DOCUMENT_ROOT'}/www/data/moodexample.txt");
print INFO "$v00, $v01, $v02, $v03, $v04, $v05, $v06,
    $v07, $v08, $v09, $v10 \n";
close (INFO);
```

Doing so would allow us to extract each response, give it a variable name within the script, and save those new local variables to the data file.

> **Note.** If you've typed something wrong in the Perl script, it is unlikely that the program will operate correctly. In fact, more often than not, the file simply will not run and you'll get an error message in your browser window. These error messages are not very helpful for the purposes of identifying the error in your code. See Chapter 15 for some tips on how to identify and fix problems in your Perl code.

EXAMPLE 2: TIME STAMPING A SUBMISSION

As an extension of the previous example, let's look at some commands that allow us to record the date and time of a submission.

Let's create a new script called **savedata2.pl**:

savedata2.pl

```
#!C:/perl/bin/perl.exe
use CGI;
$query = new CGI;

$v0= $query->param('v0');
$v1= $query->param('v1');
$v2= $query->param('v2');
$v3= $query->param('v3');
$v4= $query->param('v4');

($sec,$min,$hour,$mday,$mon,$year,$wday,$yday,$isdst) =
    localtime(time);

$ip= $query->remote_addr();
$ref= $query->referer();
open(INFO,
    ">>$ENV{'DOCUMENT_ROOT'}/www/data/moodexample2.txt");
print INFO "$mon/$mday/$year\, ";
print INFO "$hour:$min:$sec\, ";
print INFO "$ip, $ref, ";
print INFO "$v0, $v1, $v2, $v3, $v4 ";
print INFO "endline \n";
close (INFO);

print $query->header;
print $query->start_html(-title=>'Thank You');
print "<FONT FACE = 'arial' SIZE = '2'>Thank you for
    your participation in this research! </FONT>";
print $query->end_html;
```

(Be sure to modify the ACTION attribute of the FORM tag in your HTML document [moodsample2.htm] so that the submission of the mood data now activates the **savedata2.pl** script rather than the **savedata.pl** script.)

Let me highlight the new additions to the code and what they accomplish for us.

Time Stamp

The first addition to the original program is the following code:

```
($sec,$min,$hour,$mday,$mon,$year,$wday,$yday,$isdst) =
    localtime(time);
```

This command extracts the current time and date from the server's internal clock. When the **savedata2.pl** script is activated, several local variables are created (e.g., $sec, $min, $hour) that correspond to the time and date of the submission. Here is a listing of the variables that are created, what they represent, and how they are numerically qualified:

$sec	second (0 – 59)
$min	minute (0 – 59)
$hour	hour (24 hour time: 0 – 23)
$mday	day of the month
$mon	month (0 [January] – 11 [December])
$year	year (1900 + the value of $year equals the current year)
$wday	day of the week (0 [Sunday] – 6 [Saturday])
$yday	day of the year (1 – 365)
$isdst	Is it daylight savings time? (0 = no, 1 = yes)

We can print some of the more important parts of this information to our data file using the print command:

```
print INFO "$mon/$mday/$year, ";
print INFO "$hour:$min:$sec, ";
```

Notice that we strung the month, day of the month, and year variables along, separated by forward slashes (/) to create a date using the common U.S. notation: mm/dd/yy. For example, May 19, 2002 would be represented as 4/19/102 here. Also, we strung along the hour, minute, and second, separated by colons, in order to depict the time in a standard manner (e.g., 10:24:33). The ability to combine variables and regular text (e.g., the slashes and colons in the example above) is one of the powerful features of Perl, and we'll exploit it more in the next chapter when we design customized feedback for users.

Environmental Variables

As discussed above, when the user clicks the **Submit** button, a data packet is sent to your server that not only contains the user's responses to your questions, but also some environmental variables (e.g., the URL of the page that activated the script). All of this information is forced into the $query variable when we use the $query = new CGI command.

There are only two pieces of environmental information that you'll probably care about. The first is the **referrer**: the URL of the page from which the user submitted the data. This may be useful for keeping track of which condition a user was in, assuming there are different pages corresponding to different conditions. It is also useful for security purposes, as will be discussed in Chapter 15. This information can be extracted from the $query data using the following command:

```
$ref= $query->referer();
```

This command creates a new variable called $ref.

The second important environmental variable is the user's IP address. An IP (Internet Protocol) address is a sequence of numbers that is unique to each computer or Internet port. IP addresses can be useful for helping to determine whether a user has submitted data in the recent past. We'll discuss this problem in length in the final chapter of this book. For now, it is important to keep in mind that sometimes a user might participate in a study more than once—especially if it is interesting—within the same brief period of time. By tracking IP numbers, you can later sort through the data file to determine whether multiple submissions were received from the same computer within, say, a 10-minute period of time. The user's IP address can be extracted from the $query data using the following command:

```
$ip= $query->remote_addr();
```

This creates a new variable called $ip that contains the IP address of the user.

The following line of our program simply prints these two new variables, followed by a comma, to the data file:

```
print INFO "$ip, $ref, ";
```

LET'S SEE IT WORK

To see how this script saves the data, open your browser and go to the URL for your mood questionnaire. (Make sure that you've changed the ACTION attribute so it calls for savedata2.pl instead of savedata1.pl.) Answer the questions and then submit your data. Hit the **Back** button on your browser and submit some more data.

Now, in your text editor, open the moodexample2.txt file in your server's data directory. (Again, if you're using a web hosting service, don't forget to FTP the file from your server to your computer so you can view it.) You should see something similar to the information presented in Figure 5.1. Note that each submission was saved as a separate line in the file. Also, note that the IP address for your computer has been recorded in the file, as well as the URL for the site that called the Perl script (this should be the URL of your mood questionnaire). Finally, notice that the date and time of the submission have been recorded using the server's clock.

IMPORTING THE DATA INTO SPSS

One of the advantages of saving the data to a text file is that you can later import those data into your favorite spreadsheet or data analysis program. To illustrate how to do this, I'll work through an example in which we import data into SPSS version 10.0 for Windows. (The same general strategy should apply to any spreadsheet program.)

1. Open SPSS.

2. Open a new data file: File > Open > Data.

```
6/25/103, 14:45:16, 64.109.251.4, http://www.web-research-design.net/moodsurvey2.htm, MoodSurvey, 1, 0, 1, 0 endline
6/25/103, 14:45:20, 64.109.251.4, http://www.web-research-design.net/moodsurvey2.htm, MoodSurvey, 1, 1, 1, 0 endline
6/25/103, 14:45:27, 64.109.251.4, http://www.web-research-design.net/moodsurvey2.htm, MoodSurvey, 1, 1, 0, 1 endline
6/25/103, 14:45:32, 64.109.251.4, http://www.web-research-design.net/moodsurvey2.htm, MoodSurvey, 0, 1, 1, 0 endline
```

FIGURE 5.1. An example of what your data may look like when saved as a text (.txt) file.

3. In the pull-down menu labeled Files of Type, choose Text (*.txt).

4. Select the moodexample2.txt file. (If you're using an Apache server configured in the way described in Chapter 2, your data files will be located in data folder: C:\Program Files\Apache Group\Apache2\ htdocs\www\data\. If you're using a professional web hosting service, you will need to use your FTP program to transfer your data file from the server's data directory to your computer before opening it in SPSS.)

5. Once you select a file, a new window called the Text Import Wizard should appear. Follow the instructions and go with all the defaults. The only exception is when the following question is asked: "Which delimiters appear between variables?" In this case, choose only "comma" since we're using commas to separate different values of the variables within a row.

SUMMARY

This was a challenging chapter. However, it was probably your *first* introduction to CGI scripting. Once you're accustomed to the basics of the CGI process, the rest of the examples we work with in this book will be much clearer. Let's review some of the basic components of the CGI process, as discussed in this chapter.

1. When the user clicks the **Submit** button in his or her browser, he or she is sending your server one packet of data. Throughout this book I'll refer to this data packet as the **CGI data packet**.

2. The packet of data is processed by a CGI script. The specific script that processes the data is the one named by the ACTION attribute in the FORM tag of your web page.

3. A CGI script can be written to process data in a number of ways. In this chapter, we have studied a simple script that extracts the user's responses (as well as some environmental variables) and saves them to a data file on the server.

In addition to this big picture, there are some important details to keep in mind:

1.   Every CGI program that we'll write in this book will begin with the following three lines:

```
#!C:/perl/bin/perl.exe
use CGI;
$query = new CGI;
```

The first tells the server where the Perl executable file can be found. The second instructs the server to use the data packet that was sent from the user's browser. The third creates a local variable called $query that will contain all the content of the CGI data packet.

2.   Any time we want our CGI script to send the user some HTML code (e.g., to create a "thank you" page or to ask additional questions), we'll need to include the following code:

```
print $query->header;
print $query->start_html();
print $query->end_html;
```

The first and second lines act like <HTML> tags; the third line acts as the </HTML> tag. Any HTML code you want to send the browser must come in between the second and third lines, must be prefaced by the print command, and must be enclosed in double quotes. For example:

```
print $query->header;
print $query->start_html(-title=>'Thank You');
print "<FONT FACE = 'arial' SIZE = '2'>Thank you for
    your participation in this research! </FONT>";
print $query->end_html;
```

3.   Any time we want to write data to a text file, we need to open the data file with the following generic command:

```
open(INFO,
    ">>$ENV{'DOCUMENT_ROOT'}/www/data/filename.txt");
```

where "filename" is replaced by the name of the data file you want to create and add to. Once the data file is open, we can add information to the file by using the print command:

```
print INFO "$value, ";
```

Finally, when we're finished with the data file, we close it with the following generic command:

```
close (INFO);
```

4.   When programming in Perl, all lines of code must end with a semicolon. One of the most common programming mistakes is to forget the semicolon.

5.   All scalar variables that are created and used within a script need to be prefaced with a dollar sign (e.g., $age, $v01, $sex).

6.   You can assign any value from the submitted CGI data packet to a local variable within the CGI script by using the following generic structure:

```
$age = $query->param('v2');
```

In this example, a local variable called $age is created and assigned the value corresponding to "v2" in the CGI data packet. This command implies that v2 is the name of a variable in the HTML form.

Here is a review of some of the Perl commands that we learned in this chapter.

Perl commands	Function	Example

`#!C:/perl/bin/perl.exe`
`use CGI;`
`$query = new CGI;`
	These three lines of code should appear at the beginning of every CGI script that you write. (They won't always be necessary, but you can do no harm by always including them.) The first line is called the shebang! line, and specifies the location of **perl.exe** so the Perl code can be executed. The second line instructs the script to use information from the CGI data packet. The third line dumps that information into a catch-all variable named $query.	`#!C:/perl/bin/perl.exe`
		`use CGI;`
		`$query = new CGI;`

`$localvariable=`
`$query->param`
`('variablename');`
	This command extracts variables and their values from the CGI data packet. `$localvariable` is the local variable that is created to represent the variable within the script. `variablename` is the name of the variable that is being read from the CGI data packet (i.e., the name specified by the NAME attribute in the HTML INPUT tags).	`$v0= $query->param('v0');`
		Creates a local variable named $v0 that is set equal to the value of v0 from the CGI data packet submitted by the user.

Perl commands	Function	Example
`open(INFO, ">>c:\\filename. txt");` `print INFO "$v0 $v1 $v3 \n";` `close (INFO);`	These commands are used to open a text file, print information to the text file, and, finally, close the text file. \n creates a line break within the data file—a useful way to separate one person's data from the next person's data. INFO is a *file handle*—a short way of referring to the data file in question within the Perl script. >> tells the server to append the data to the file as opposed to overwriting what already exists in the file.	`open(INFO, ">>$ENV{'DOCUMENT_ROOT'} /www/data/ demographics.txt");` `print INFO "$name, $age, $sex \n";` `close (INFO);` In this example, the values of the local variables $name, $age, and $sex are saved to the data file called demographics.txt on the server. The use of commas between variables has the effect of inserting commas between values in the text file, making it a "comma-delimited" text file—one that is easily imported into Microsoft Excel, S-Plus, or SPSS.
`print $query-> header;` `print $query-> start_html (-title=>'Thank You');` `print $query-> end_html;`	The first two lines are used to send HTML information to a browser from a CGI script and specify the title of the web page. They function much like an <HTML> tag in an HTML document. The third line functions as a </HTML> tag. These lines must be included any time HTML information is sent to the browser from a CGI script.	`print $query->header;` `print $query->start_html (-title=>'Thank You');` `print "<FONT FACE = 'arial' SIZE = '2'>Thank you for your participation in this research! </FONT>";` `print $query->end_html;`
`print "text";`	The print command is used to print information to a text file or to the user's browser. To print the information to the browser as HTML code, the codes discussed above must be used first. To print the information to a text file, the text file must be open and the file handle must be specified (see open above).	Printing HTML code to the browser: `print $query->header;` `print $query->start_html (-title=>'Menu');` `print "<FONT FACE = 'arial' SIZE = '2'>Welcome to the menu page. </FONT>";` `print $query->end_html;` Printing information to a text file: `open(INFO, ">>$ENV{'DOCUMENT_ROOT'} /www/data/mydata.txt");` `print INFO "$name, $age, $sex \n";` `close (INFO);`
`$variable`	Scalar variables are represented in Perl with a dollar sign followed by the name of the variable. Use the equal sign to assign a value to a local variable within a Perl script.	`$name = "Chris";` This creates a local variable called $name and assigns it the value Chris.

Perl commands	Function	Example
`@array`	Arrays are represented in Perl with a @ sign followed by the name of the variable. Arrays are composed of multiple values. The first element of an array is indexed as the 0th element.	`@names = ("chris", "caroline", "bumpy");` This creates an array called @names consisting of three names. `$names[2] = "spappy";` This assigns the 2nd element of the array @names the value spappy.
`localtime(time);`	This code extracts the current time and date from the server's clock	`($sec,$min,$hour,$mday,$mon, $year,$wday,$yday,$isdst) = localtime(time);` This code extracts the current time and date from the server's clock and saves the different pieces of information as local variables.
`$query->referer();`	The referrer command extracts the URL of the web page that activated the CGI script.	`$ref= $query->referer();` This code extracts the URL and assigns its value to a local variable named $ref.
`$query-> remote_addr();`	The remote address command extracts the IP address of the computer that submitted the CGI data packet.	`$ip= $query->remote_addr();` This code extracts the IP address of the user and assigns its value to a local variable named $ip.
`flock(filehandle, 2);`	Locks a data file so that it can only be accessed by one user (or one CGI script) at a time. The "2" instructs the server to request exclusive access. The data file will be unlocked automatically once the writing process is complete. The file writing process is usually very quick, so it is highly unlikely that two users will "bump into" one another in the data writing process.	`flock(INFO, 2);`

Chapter 6

Providing Customized Feedback to Research Participants

One of the most valuable features of using the Internet for conducting behavioral research is that it allows us, through interactivity with the user, to provide more information to our research participants than they would normally obtain in a traditional study. Specifically, you can create a CGI script that analyses the user's responses and explains to the user what those responses might mean. You can also program the script to analyze the results from other users and provide the current user with information about his or her responses in comparison to those of others. This kind of feedback can make the research experience much more personal and rewarding for the participant. Moreover, your research participants will probably be much more intrinsically motivated to participate in your research (and to do so conscientiously) if they know they are going to learn something interesting *about themselves*.

In this chapter we're going to focus on analyzing a participant's responses and providing him or her with instantaneous feedback. We will illustrate this technique by creating an Internet questionnaire designed to measure self-esteem and a corresponding CGI script that processes the responses and gives the user a summary of his or her self-esteem scores. Although we will be focusing on a specific application in this chapter, the techniques and skills underlying this application can be used in a variety of research contexts.

This chapter is substantially more complex than the previous ones, and it may take a bit of experimenting and a second reading before some of the basic commands and strategies begin to feel intuitive. If certain aspects of the programming commands or logic seem obtuse at first, don't give up. Read through the chapter once, work though the exercises, try experimenting with the code a bit, and then reread the chapter again. Once you've mastered the skills taught in this chapter, you will have cleared a substantial hurdle, and you should be able to imagine how many of the techniques discussed here can be used in other creative ways.

PROVIDING FEEDBACK: AVERAGING A USER'S RESPONSES

To illustrate the technique of creating customized feedback, let's create a web page designed to measure a person's self esteem. The Rosenberg Self-Esteem Inventory is a commonly used self-report instrument for assessing self-esteem in adults (Blascovich & Tomaka, 1993; Rosenberg, 1965). For simplicity, let's use the first 5 items of this 10-item scale.

We'll need to create two files. The first will be an HTML file for the questionnaire per se. The second will be a CGI script for processing the data. Copy the HTML code below to a blank document in your text editor. (Recall that these scripts can be copied-and-pasted from the web page for this book at http://www.web-research-design.net/). Save the file as **self-esteem.htm** in the **Public HTML** directory on your server.

self-esteem.htm

```
<HTML>
<TITLE>Self-Esteem Test</TITLE>
<FONT FACE = 'arial' SIZE = '2'>
<B>This page is designed to assess your self-
    esteem.</B><BR> <BR>
Please answer the following questions. Once you have
    answered each question, click the button labeled
```

```
<I> calculate my score.</I> The web page will then
calculate your self-esteem score, and tell you more
about how you compare to others.<BR><BR>

<FORM ACTION = '/cgi-bin/self-esteem.pl' METHOD =
    'post'>

1. I feel that I'm a person of worth, at least on an
    equal plane with others.<BR>
Strongly Disagree
<INPUT TYPE = 'radio' NAME = 'v01' VALUE = '1'>
<INPUT TYPE = 'radio' NAME = 'v01' VALUE = '2'>
<INPUT TYPE = 'radio' NAME = 'v01' VALUE = '3'>
<INPUT TYPE = 'radio' NAME = 'v01' VALUE = '4'>
<INPUT TYPE = 'radio' NAME = 'v01' VALUE = '5'>
Strongly Agree<BR><BR>

2. I feel that I have a number of good qualities.<BR>
Strongly Disagree
<INPUT TYPE = 'radio' NAME = 'v02' VALUE = '1'>
<INPUT TYPE = 'radio' NAME = 'v02' VALUE = '2'>
<INPUT TYPE = 'radio' NAME = 'v02' VALUE = '3'>
<INPUT TYPE = 'radio' NAME = 'v02' VALUE = '4'>
<INPUT TYPE = 'radio' NAME = 'v02' VALUE = '5'>
Strongly Agree<BR><BR>

3. All in all, I am inclined to feel that I am a
    failure.<BR>
Strongly Disagree
<INPUT TYPE = 'radio' NAME = 'v03' VALUE = '1'>
<INPUT TYPE = 'radio' NAME = 'v03' VALUE = '2'>
<INPUT TYPE = 'radio' NAME = 'v03' VALUE = '3'>
<INPUT TYPE = 'radio' NAME = 'v03' VALUE = '4'>
<INPUT TYPE = 'radio' NAME = 'v03' VALUE = '5'>
Strongly Agree<BR><BR>

4. I am able to do things as well as most other
    people.
<BR>
Strongly Disagree
<INPUT TYPE = 'radio' NAME = 'v04' VALUE = '1'>
<INPUT TYPE = 'radio' NAME = 'v04' VALUE = '2'>
<INPUT TYPE = 'radio' NAME = 'v04' VALUE = '3'>
<INPUT TYPE = 'radio' NAME = 'v04' VALUE = '4'>
<INPUT TYPE = 'radio' NAME = 'v04' VALUE = '5'>
Strongly Agree<BR><BR>
```

```
5. I feel I do not have much to be proud of.
<BR>
Strongly Disagree
<INPUT TYPE = 'radio' NAME = 'v05' VALUE = '1'>
<INPUT TYPE = 'radio' NAME = 'v05' VALUE = '2'>
<INPUT TYPE = 'radio' NAME = 'v05' VALUE = '3'>
<INPUT TYPE = 'radio' NAME = 'v05' VALUE = '4'>
<INPUT TYPE = 'radio' NAME = 'v05' VALUE = '5'>
Strongly Agree<BR><BR><BR>

<INPUT TYPE = 'submit' VALUE = 'Calculate my score'>
</FORM></FONT></HTML>
```

Next, enter the URL for the page in the address bar of your browser. On my server, the appropriate URL for the page is http://www.web-research-design. net/self-esteem.htm. The corresponding web page is illustrated in Figure 6.1. Feel free to begin answering some of the questions, but do not press the **Submit** button yet.

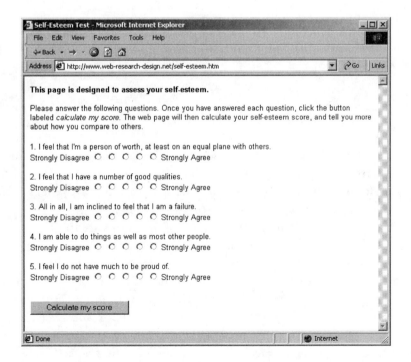

FIGURE 6.1. This page illustrates a simple, five-item self-esteem scale.

Next, we want to create a CGI script that will (1) compute the user's average self-esteem score on the five items and (2) tell the user what his or her average score is. Copy the following code to a blank document in your text editor and save the file as self-esteem.pl in the cgi-bin directory of your server.

self-esteem.pl

```
#!C:/perl/bin/perl.exe
use CGI;
$query = new CGI;

$v01= $query->param('v01');
$v02= $query->param('v02');
$v03= $query->param('v03');
$v04= $query->param('v04');
$v05= $query->param('v05');

$esteem = ($v01 + $v02 + (6 - $v03) + $v04 + (6 -
   $v05) ) /5;
$esteem2 = sprintf("%.2f", $esteem);

print $query->header;
print $query->start_html(-title=>'Thank You');
print "<FONT FACE = 'arial' SIZE = '2'><B>Self-Esteem
   Results Page</B><BR><BR>
Your self-esteem score is a $esteem2, on a scale
   ranging from 1 to 5.
</FONT>";
print $query->end_html;
```

Once both files are present on your server, go ahead and play around with the self-esteem web page a bit (i.e., answer the questions and submit the data) in order to get a feel for what is happening. Now, let's break the code apart in order to see how the program works.

Notice that the first three lines of this script are the same three lines that come at the beginning of any CGI script. Also, notice that the next block contains commands that are similar to those we used in the last chapter. These commands are designed to extract the values associated with the variables called v01, v02, v03, v04, and v05 from $query and assign them to local variables named $v01, $v02, $v03, $v04, and $v05, respectively.

The next line creates a local variable named $esteem. This variable will be equal to the average of the responses to the five self-esteem items:

```
$esteem = ($v01 + $v02 + (6 - $v03) + $v04 + (6 -
   $v05) ) /5;
```

To give you a concrete sense of what is happening in this command line, let's assume that the user has provided the following responses to the five self-esteem items: 5, 5, 1, 5, and 1. If so, the local variables that we've created will take on the following values: $v01 = 5, $v02 = 5, $v03 = 1, $v04 = 5, and $v05 = 1.

If we place these values in the equation printed above, we obtain

$(5 + 5 + (6 - 1) + 5 + (6 - 1)) / 5$

or

$(5 + 5 + 5 + 5 + 5)/5 = 5$

Thus, the variable $esteem will equal 5 for this subject.

Note. Items 3 and 5 are called **reverse keyed** items in survey research because they are worded in the opposite direction of the construct being assessed. Thus, a *low* response to an item such as "I hate myself" is indicative of *high* self-esteem. When we average the self-esteem scores, we need to reverse key the responses to these items so that high values map onto low values and vice versa. The most efficient way to do this is to subtract from the reverse keyed items 1 plus the highest possible response option. In this example, 1 plus the highest value of 5, is 6.

Note. You can use a variety of mathematical expressions in Perl. Here is a list of some of the common operations you might need to use:

Operation	Perl symbol	Example
addition	+	$x + $y (adds the values of $x and $y)
subtraction	–	$x - $y (subtracts the value of $y from $x)
multiplication	*	$x * $y (multiplies the values of $x and $y)
division	/	$x/$y (divides the value of $y into $x)
exponent	**	$x**2 (raises $x to the second power)
square root	**(.5)	$x**(.5) (raises $x to the .5 power—the square root)

Creating mathematical expressions in Perl is quite simple. Let's assume, for example, that we have three variables, $x1, $x2, and $x3, and we want to average them and assign the average to a variable called $average. The following expression will accomplish this: $average = ($x1 + $x2 + $x3)/3; This line of code translates to, "Take the sum of the values contained in $x1, $x2, and $x3, divide this sum by 3, and assign that value—an average—to the variable $average." Notice that we placed the terms we wanted to sum within parentheses. We need to do this because, although Perl follows the basic order of mathematical operations and executes multiplication and division before addition and subtraction, it executes operations grouped within parentheses first. If we had omitted the parentheses and instead typed $average = $x1 + $x2 + $x3/3, Perl would have divided 3 into the value of $x3 and then added that value to $x1 and $x2.

The next line creates a new variable called $esteem2. This variable will contain the value of $esteem rounded to two decimal places. If we wanted to round this variable to four decimal places, we could use the following command: `$esteem2 = sprintf("%.4f", $esteem);`

The next set of commands should be familiar to you. As we saw in the last chapter, these commands are responsible for sending HTML code to the user's browser. What is particularly noteworthy here is that we are able to insert a variable, $esteem2, into the HTML code, and Perl automatically *substitutes* the value of that variable into the text. This is a highly useful feature of Perl because it allows us to tailor the contents of the web page to the user. This process of **substitution** is critical for creating dynamic web pages in Perl.

PROVIDING FEEDBACK: AVERAGING A USER'S RESPONSES AND SAVING THE DATA

Now, let's combine the skills we just acquired with those learned in the last chapter. Specifically, let's compute the user's self-esteem level and save it to a data file on our server. Let's begin by modifying our original HTML document. Open **self-esteem.htm** in your text editor and replace the line

```
<FORM ACTION = '/cgi-bin/self-esteem.pl' METHOD =
    'post'>
```

with

self-esteem2.htm

```
<FORM ACTION = '/cgi-bin/self-esteem2.pl' METHOD =
   'post'>
```

Save the modified HTML document as **self-esteem2.htm** in your Public HTML directory. Create a new document in your text editor and copy the following code to the document. Save the file as **self-esteem2.pl** to the cgi-bin directory of your server.

self-esteem2.pl

```
#!C:/perl/bin/perl.exe
use CGI;
$query = new CGI;

$v01= $query->param('v01');
$v02= $query->param('v02');
$v03= $query->param('v03');
$v04= $query->param('v04');
$v05= $query->param('v05');
$esteem = ($v01 + $v02 + (6 - $v03) + $v04 + (6 -
   $v05) ) /5;

$esteem2 = sprintf("%.2f", $esteem);
($sec,$min,$hour,$mday,$mon,$year,$wday,$yday,$isdst) =
   localtime(time);

$ip= $query->remote_addr();

open(INFO,
   ">>$ENV{'DOCUMENT_ROOT'}/www/data/selfesteem.txt");
print INFO "$mon/$mday/$year\, ";
print INFO "$hour:$min:$sec\, ";
print INFO "$ip, ";
print INFO "$v01, $v02, $v03, $v04, $v05,";
print INFO "$esteem2, ";
print INFO "endline \n";
close (INFO);

print $query->header;
print $query->start_html(-title=>'Thank You');

print "<FONT FACE = 'arial' SIZE = '2'><B>Self-Esteem
   Results Page</B><BR><BR>
Your self-esteem score is $esteem2, on a scale
   ranging from 1 to 5.
</FONT>";

print $query->end_html;
```

This script, in addition to providing our user with his or her average self-esteem score, saves the user's data to a file. Specifically, we've added the date, time, the user's IP address, the user's responses to each of the five questions, and the user's average self-esteem score to a data file called self-esteem.txt. To accomplish this, we've simply lifted the code discussed in the previous chapter and inserted it here. The only new thing we've done is that, in addition to saving the user's responses, we've also saved his or her average self-esteem score, which was calculated within the script (print INFO "$esteem2, ";). Play around with the web page a bit on your server and open the self-esteem.txt file from your server's **data** directory in your text editor. You should see that the data have been recorded.

DATA ANALYSIS ON THE SERVER: AVERAGING THE RESPONSES OF EVERYONE IN YOUR SAMPLE

Now that you've seen a simple example of how we can take the user's input and perform computations on it, let's make the program a bit more sophisticated. What we're going to do next is modify the program so that, in addition to providing the user his or her self-esteem score, it tells the user what the average score is for people in our sample. This will require instructing the server to open the self-esteem.txt data file, read the existing data, and compute an average. Copy the following code and save it as self-esteem3.pl in you server's **cgi-bin** directory.

self-esteem3.pl

```
#!C:/perl/bin/perl.exe
use CGI;
$query = new CGI;

$v01= $query->param('v01');
$v02= $query->param('v02');
$v03= $query->param('v03');
$v04= $query->param('v04');
$v05= $query->param('v05');

$esteem = ($v01 + $v02 + (6 - $v03) + $v04 + (6 -
    $v05) ) /5;
$esteem2 = sprintf("%.2f", $esteem);
```

```perl
($sec,$min,$hour,$mday,$mon,$year,$wday,$yday,$isdst) =
   localtime(time);

$ip= $query->remote_addr();

open(INFO, ">>$ENV{'DOCUMENT_ROOT'}/www/data/self-
   esteem.txt");
print INFO "$mon/$mday/$year\, ";
print INFO "$hour:$min:$sec\, ";
print INFO "$ip, ";
print INFO "$v01, $v02, $v03, $v04, $v05,";
print INFO "$esteem2, ";
print INFO "endline \n";
close (INFO);

$sum= 0;
$n= 0;

open(INFO, "$ENV{'DOCUMENT_ROOT'}/www/data/self-
   esteem.txt");
@data = <INFO>;
close(INFO);

foreach $key (@data)
{
($adate,$atime,$aip,$av01,$av02,$av03,$av04,$av05,$aeste
   em2,$aendline)=split(/,/,$key);
$sum= $sum + $aesteem2;
$n= $n + 1;
}

$esteemmean= $sum/$n;
$esteemmean = sprintf("%.2f", $esteemmean);

print $query->header;
print $query->start_html(-title=>'Thank You');
print "<FONT FACE = 'arial' SIZE = '2'><B>Self-Esteem
   Results Page</B><BR><BR>
Your self-esteem score is $esteem2, on a scale
   ranging from 1 to 5.<BR><BR>
The average self-esteem score for people who have
   taken this survey is $esteemmean.<BR><BR>
To date, $n people have taken this survey.
</FONT>";
print $query->end_html;
```

Also, just for simplicity, edit your **self-esteem2.htm** file so that it directs the submitted data to **self-esteem3.pl** instead of **self-esteem2.pl**. Save the modified file as **self-esteem3.htm** in your **Public HTML** directory.

self-esteem3.htm

We're working with the same code that we used before, but with some new additions. I'll explain these additions below, but not necessarily in the same order in which they appear in the code. Here is the first significant change:

```
open(INFO, "$ENV{'DOCUMENT_ROOT'}/www/data/self-
   esteem.txt");
@data = <INFO>;
close(INFO);
```

This set of commands translates to, "Open the data file called **self-esteem.txt** in the server's **data** folder, assign the contents of this file to an array called @data, then close the data file." We will now have a local array called @data that contains all the information in our data file. (Please see the Note on the distinction between scalar variables and array variables in Chapter 5.)

Here is the next set of commands:

```
foreach $key (@data)
{
($adate,$atime,$aip,$av01,$av02,$av03,$av04,$av05,
   $aesteem2,$aendline)=split(/,/,$key);
}
```

The **foreach** command is used to execute a set of commands (those between the braces) repetitively. A set of commands that are carried out repeatedly by a few lines of code is called a **loop**. We'll discuss two kinds of loops in this book, the foreach loop (which we are using here for the first time) and the **for-next** loop (which we will discuss in the next chapter). This block of code translates to, "For each line of data contained in the array named @data, split the information into distinct values called $adate, $atime, . . . $aendline based on the occurrence of a comma." As a result, the program will cycle or loop through each row in the data file and perform operations within each row. ($key is a temporary label used to reference each line of data as it is extracted from @data.) The split command instructs the server to separate information appearing on the same line of the data file into distinct elements. In this example, it makes those distinctions on the basis of commas.

Whenever a comma appears, the program will assume that one variable has ended and a new one is beginning.

Note. In the **split** command, we've surrounded the comma with slashes: /,/. As you have seen, commas (and double quotes) are commonly used in Perl. Whenever we want a comma to refer to something in particular (i.e., a piece of information in a response or text file), rather than to refer to part of the Perl programming code per se, we surround it with slashes. This tells Perl to treat the comma as a real piece of information as opposed to a piece of programming code.

Within the foreach loop, we also included the following two lines of code:

```
$sum= $sum + $aesteem2;
$n= $n + 1;
```

These two lines are responsible for aggregating information from the data file. In particular, when the program begins, we create two variables, $sum and $n, and set them equal to zero:

```
$sum= 0;
$n= 0;
```

As the foreach routine reads each line of data from the file, however, it will increment the values of $sum and $n. Specifically, it will take the value of $aesteem2 from the current line in the data file and add it to the variable $sum. In the case of $n, each time we process a line of the @data array, we add 1 to the current value of $n. We'll be using this incrementing strategy a lot in CGI programming, so let's discuss exactly what is happening in a bit more detail.

Let's assume the data file looks like this:

```
4/22/102, 18:34:33, 131.193.133.59, 5, 5, 1, 5, 1,
   5.00, endline
4/22/102, 18:34:48, 131.193.133.59, 2, 4, 2, 4, 2,
   3.60, endline
4/22/102, 18:35:4, 131.193.133.59, 5, 4, 1, 4, 2,
   4.40, endline
```

A new user completes the questionnaire and clicks the **Submit** button. Before the foreach loop begins, we set $n and $sum to zero. The first time we enter the foreach loop, we split the first line of @data into distinct variables called $adate, $atime, . . . $aendline. The first time through the loop, these variables will represent the values for the first participant. The variable $aesteem2, for example, represents the first participant's self-esteem score (i.e., 5.00).

Note. We're going to give these values different names than those used before. Names such as $v01, for example, represent the *current* user's response to question 1. Because $v01 already represents a value of interest locally within the program, we don't want to copy over it by assigning the first participant's response to question 1 to the same variable name. Instead, we use a different name, such as $av01.

Next, we take the value of $aesteem2 and add it to the current value of $sum. Because $sum equals 0 when we first begin the loop, the `$sum + $aesteem2` operation is equivalent to 0 + 5.00. Now, $sum will equal 5.00. Next, we take the current value of $n, which is zero, and add 1 to it: `$n + 1` or 0 + 1 Now, $n equals 1. We have now executed all the commands within the loop, so we go back to the beginning of the foreach loop and operate on the second line of data in the @data array.

The program will perform the operations again, but on the second line of data in @data. Specifically, it will break the second line of data in @data into distinct variables. Because it is using the same variable names as it did before, it will copy over the values from the first participant. For example, the second time through the loop, $aesteem2 will equal 3.60 instead of 5.00.

Next, the program increments the values of $sum and $n. Because $sum currently equals 5.00, we add 3.60 to 5.00, giving us 8.60. In other words, the program has added the current value of $aesteem2 to $sum. We also increment $n. Because n$ is now equal to 1, by executing `$n= $n + 1` the computer is adding 1 to 1, yielding 2. Thus, as the program finishes its second run through the loop, $sum equals 8.60 and $n equals 2.

In the third and final time through the loop, the program will do the same operations again. It splits the third line of data in @data into distinct values, copying over the values that were previously represented by $adate, $aip, and so on. The value represented by $aseteem2 now corresponds to the third participant's self-esteem score: 4.40. We add this value to $sum, yielding 8.60 + 4.40 or 13.00. We also increment $n by 1, so $n now equals 3.

Because there are no more lines of data in the @data array, the foreach loop ends, and the server moves on to the next line of code in **self-esteem3.pl**. Notice that what we now have a local variable, $sum, that is equal to the sum of everyone's self-esteem scores. We also have a local variable called $n that contains the sample size. By dividing $sum by $n, we can compute the average self-esteem score of the sample. The next two lines accomplish this operation:

```
$esteemmean = $sum/$n;
$esteemmean = sprintf("%.2f", $esteemmean);
```

The new variable, $esteemmean, will equal $sum/$n—the average self-esteem score in the sample. We then round that value to two decimal places yielding 4.33.

We have covered *a lot* thus far, so let's review what we have learned before we continue. With **self-esteem3.htm** and **self-esteem3.pl**, we've instructed the server to read the data in the self-esteem file—the file that contains all the information we've collected from our research participants to date. Using a foreach loop, we've extracted each person's self-esteem score, and added that value to a variable called $sum. This allows us to add all the self-esteem scores in the sample. Also, each time we went through the loop, we added 1 to the value of $n. Doing so allowed us to calculate the sample size. Finally, once we went through each line of data in our file, we computed the sample mean by dividing $sum by $n.

Finally, notice that we've included the variable $esteemmean in the HTML code we send to the user. The user learns not only what his or her self-esteem score is, but also what the average self-esteem score is for people in the sample. The server has analyzed the data in your sample and reported the results to your participant.

USING IF–ELSE CONDITIONALS TO TAILOR THE FEEDBACK FURTHER

Let's go one step further and tell our participant whether his or her score is higher or lower than the sample mean. We can do so by replacing the HTML commands at the end of **self-esteem3.pl** with those listed below. Save the modified document as **self-esteem4.pl** in your **cgi-bin** directory. Also, to make it easier to keep track, revise your **self-esteem3.htm** document so that, when the data are submitted, the **self-esteem4.pl** script is activated. Save the modified file as **self-esteem4.htm** in your **Public HTML** folder.

self-esteem4.htm

self-esteem4.pl

```
print $query->header;
print $query->start_html(-title=>'Thank You');
print "<FONT FACE = 'arial' SIZE = '2'><B>Self-Esteem
   Results Page</B><BR><BR>
Your self-esteem score is $esteem2, on a scale
   ranging from 1 to 5.<BR><BR>
The average self-esteem score for people who have
   taken this survey is $esteemmean.<BR>";

if($esteem > $esteemmean){
print "Your self-esteem is higher than that of the
   average participant.";
}

if($esteem < $esteemmean){
print "Your self-esteem is lower than that of the
   average participant.";
}

print "<BR><BR>To date, $n people have taken this
   survey.<BR></FONT>";
print $query->end_html;
```

The following set of commands are enclosed in what is called an **if–else** logical condition.

```
if ($esteem > $esteemmean) { }
```

When the program sees the "if" command, it determines whether the conditions outlined within parentheses have been met. If so, it executes the commands contained within braces. If not, then it skips over the commands in braces. We're using these if-else conditionals to customize the feedback the user receives. The conditionals in this script roughly translate to: "If the value of $esteem is greater than the value of $esteemmean, print the following line: 'Your self-esteem is higher than that of the average participant.' If the value of

$esteem is less than the value of $esteemmean, then print the following line: 'Your self-esteem is lower than that of the average participant.' "

As shown in Figure 6.2, only one of these two lines will be printed for the user. The conditionals are set up in a mutually exclusive manner: The user's self-esteem can't be simultaneously higher *and* lower than the average score in the sample. If the user's self-esteem level is exactly equal to the sample mean, neither condition will be met, and nothing new will be printed for the user.

In the example above, we used an "if" condition to determine whether $esteem was greater than $esteeemmean and another "if" condition to determine whether $esteem was less than $esteemmean. We could have also used an "else" condition, coupled with an "if" condition, to accomplish this task.

```
if($esteem > $esteemmean){
print "Your self-esteem is higher than that of the
   average participant.";
}
else{
print "Your self-esteem is lower than or equal to
   that of the average participant.";
}
```

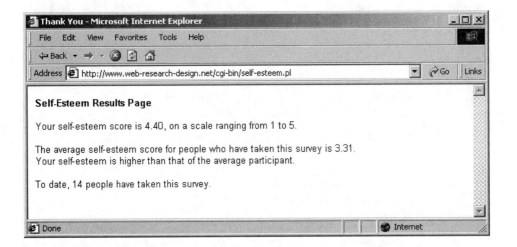

FIGURE 6.2. The CGI script averages the user's responses to provide him or her with a single self-esteem score and also summarizes for the user the data of previous users saved in the text file.

In this case, the user receives the first piece of feedback if his or her self-esteem score is higher than that of the average user. If this condition is not satisfied, the program executes the commands within the braces following the "else" statement and the user is told that his or her self-esteem score is lower than or equal to that of the typical participant.

The use of if-else conditionals is a valuable way to control the flow of operations in a program. In fact, you'll probably find the if-else methodology one of the most useful available as you begin to design your own Internet research studies. We've used it here to determine what kind of feedback the participant receives. You'll see many more examples of the use of if-else conditionals in the rest of this book.

Note. There are a number of **logical conditions** that can be tested with both numeric and text-based information within an if-else command. Here are some common logical conditions that are used with **numbers**:

Condition	Logical Test
$x is equal to $y	if($x == $y){}
$x does not equal $y	if($x != $y){}
$x is greater than $y	if($x > $y){}
$x is less than $y	if($x < $y){}
$x is less than or equal to $y	if($x <= $y){}
$x is greater than or equal to $y	if($x >= $y){}
The and conjunction	if($x == $y && $x != 0){}

(This allows you to test two logical conditions simultaneously. In order for this logical condition to be true, both conditions must be met.)

The or conjunction	if($x == $y || $x != 0){}

(This allows you to test two logical conditions simultaneously. In order for this logical condition to be true, at least one of the conditions must be met.)

Logical conditions may also be tested with **strings**—a sequence of characters (alphabetical, numeric, or symbolic). For example, if a user typed in a password, we might want to test that against what we know to be the user's password, based on our data base. In this case, we want to know whether the user's response, $x, is equal to the stored password, $y. Here are some common logical conditions that are tested with strings.

Condition	Logical Test
$x is equal to $y	`if($x eq $y){}`
$x does not equal $y	`if($x ne $y){}`
$x is greater than $y	`if($x gt $y){}`
$x is less than $y	`if($x lt $y){}`
$x is less than or equal to $y	`if($x le $y){}`
$x is greater than or equal to $y	`if($x ge $y){}`
The and conjunction	`if($x eq $y && $x ne $z){}`

(This allows you to test two logical conditions simultaneously. In order for this logical condition to be true, both conditions must be met.)

| The or conjunction | `if($x eq $y || $x ne $z){}` |

(This allows you to test two logical conditions simultaneously. In order for this logical condition to be true, at least one of the conditions must be met.)

It is not necessary that the tests be performed on local variables; actual text could be used too. For example, we could perform the following test: `if($x eq "happy")`. In this example we have included the word happy in quotes because it is a string and not a numeric value. When strings are being used in their literal forms vs. their variable or representational forms (e.g., "happy" vs. $y), they need to be enclosed in double quotes.

SAMPLE SIZE AND FEEDBACK

If there are only a handful of participants in your study, the average self-esteem score that you compute will be statistically unstable (i.e., the average score may change a lot each time a new person participates in the study), and it is not prudent to provide the user with feedback based on an unstable statistic.

There are at least two ways around this problem. First, if you're dealing with a well-studied subject, such as self-esteem, it would be easy to find out what the average self-esteem score is in other samples, and use that value instead of one estimated from your (for now) small sample. Let's assume that the average self-esteem score in other samples tends to be 4.2. We could add the following line of code to our CGI program, right before the `print $query->header` line:

```
if($n < 30){
$esteemmean= 4.2;
}
```

Now, if the sample size is less than 30, the program will change the value of $esteemmean to 4.2. If the sample size is greater than or equal to 30, it will use the actual sample mean that was computed from your data file.

Another solution is to not report sample information when the sample size is small. Here we use an if-else statement that only prints information about the sample average if the sample size is larger than 30.

```
print $query->header;
print $query->start_html(-title=>'Thank You');
print "<FONT FACE = 'arial' SIZE = '2'><B>Self-Esteem
    Results Page</B><BR><BR>
Your self-esteem score is $esteem2, on a scale
    ranging from 1 to 5.<BR><BR>";

if($n > 30){
print "The average self-esteem score for people who
    have taken this survey is $esteemmean.<BR><BR>
To date, $n people have taken this survey.";

if($esteem > $esteemmean){
print "Your self-esteem is higher than that of the
    average participant.";
}

if($esteem < $esteemmean){
print "Your self-esteem is lower than that of the
    average participant.";
}

}

print "</FONT>";
print $query->end_html;
```

> **Note.** In this code, we have nested some if-else conditionals (i.e., those concerning whether to print information about being above or below the sample mean) within another if-else conditional (i.e., that concerning whether or not to print information about the sample mean). Nesting can be a very useful tool, but you need to make sure that all opening brackets have been closed or your program will not run correctly.

SUMMARY

In this chapter we've covered a lot of territory! In the process of learning how to provide our participants with informative feedback about their responses, we learned a variety of generic Perl skills, such as how to (1) read data from a text file into an array of variables that can be manipulated easily, (2) create simple foreach loops to process each line of data from a text file, (3) use if-then conditions to tailor feedback in specific ways, and (4) insert customized variables, such as a user's self-esteem score, into the HTML code that is passed from our server to the user's browser. Let's revisit each of these points before moving on to the next chapter.

1. To read data from an already existing text file on the server, use the following generic commands:

```
open(INFO,
    "$ENV{'DOCUMENT_ROOT'}/www/data/datafile.txt");
@data = <INFO>;
close(INFO);
```

This code translates to, "open the text file called datafile.txt in the data folder on the server, take contents of that file and assign it to an array named @data, and, finally, close the data file."

2. We can process the data we've already extracted from a text file by cycling though the data line-by-line (i.e., person-by-person or row-by-row) using the foreach command.

```
foreach $key (@data)
{
($adate,$atime,$aip,$av01,$av02,$av03,$av04,$av05,
    $aesteem2,$aendline)=split(/,/,$key);
$sum = $sum + $aesteem2;
}
```

This code, for example, takes the information from the array named @data and, for each line of data, splits the line into separate variables, dividing it at each comma in the line. The values are assigned temporarily to local variables, such as $adate and $av03. In this code, the variable $aesteem2 is added to the variable $sum for each line of data. Thus, each time we loop through the array, we add that person's self-esteem score to the sum of the previous self-esteem scores.

3.   To tailor responses to the user we use if-then conditions. For example, the following code, in braces, will only be executed by the server if the value of $n is greater than 40:

```
if($n > 40){
print "The sample size is larger than 40.";
}
```

4.   We can customize the feedback the user receives by *substituting* Perl variables into the HTML code that we send to the user. For example, if the value of $average is 5.43, the code `print "The average score is $average";` will print, "The average score is 5.43" instead of literally printing "The average score is $average." Perl understands that you intend for it to substitute the *value* of the variable $average rather than, literally, the name of the variable. This is one of the most powerful features of CGI programming in Perl.

Here is a review of the Perl commands that were introduced in this chapter.

Perl commands	Function	Example
`sprintf("%.Xf", $variable);`	This command can be used to round a variable to X decimal places.	`$esteem2 = sprintf("%.4f", $esteem);` (This rounds the value of $esteem to four decimal places, and names the result $esteem.2)
`open(INFO, "ENV{'DOCUMENT_ROOT'} /www/data/textfile. txt");` `@array = <INFO>;` `close(INFO);`	This set of commands opens a text file, extracts the information to an array, and then closes the text file. INFO is a file handle that is used to temporarily reference the contents of the file.	`open(INFO, "ENV{'DOCUMENT_ROOT'} /www/data/mydata.txt");` `@data = <INFO>;` `close(INFO);` (This example opens a text file called **mydata.txt** and dumps the contents into an array named @data. The data can then be manipulated within the script by manipulating the array @data.)

Perl commands	Function	Example

`foreach $key (@array)`
`{`
`($variable01,`
`$variable02,`
`$variable03) =`
`split(/,/,$key);`
`}`
	The foreach command is used in this context to construct a loop that cycles through each line of data within an array. $key is a temporary label used to reference each line of data in the array as it is processed. How the elements are processed is specified within braces.
	The split command is used to specify the way elements within a row will be partitioned into discrete variables.
		`foreach $key (@data)`
		`{`
		`($v01, $v02, $v03) =`
		`split(/,/,$key);`
		`$sum = $sum + $v02;`
		`}`
		(In this example, each row of information in @data is separately partitioned into three variables. Each time through the loop, the second variable, $v02, is added to $sum. This allows the programmer to add together all the values of $v02 in the data set.)

`if(condition){}`
`else {}`
	The if-else command is used to control the flow of operations within a script. The commands within braces are only executed if the conditions within parentheses are met. If the conditions are not met, the commands within the else braces are executed.	`if($n < 30){`
		`$esteemmean= 4.2;`
		`}`
		`else{`
		`$esteemmean = 3.2;`
		`}`
		(In this example, the value of $esteemmean is set to 4.2 if the value of $n is less than 30). If this condition is not met, then the commands within the else braces are executed.

Chapter 7

Randomizing the Order of Stimuli

From a research design perspective, the self-esteem survey we created in the previous chapters has a minor limitation. Specifically, the items were always presented in the same order. The item "I feel that I'm a person of worth, at least on an equal plane with others," for example, always came first, whereas "I feel I do not have much to be proud of" always came last. When research stimuli are presented in the same order for all participants, we introduce the possibility that there might be subtle effects having to do with a particular order of questions that might contaminate our results. Although these kinds of effects might not be problematic for some studies, it should be clear that there are other research contexts (e.g., those that require a repeated-measures design) where using the same presentation order across participants could seriously undermine the inferences the researcher could draw from the data.

One way of dealing with this problem is to randomize the presentation order of stimuli whenever possible. It would be difficult to do this with a normal HTML web page. Each user, arriving at an HTML page, will see the same page—with the items in the same order. It is possible, however, to program a CGI script to deliver the stimuli in a random fashion.

In this chapter we're going to take advantage of the fact that CGI scripts can be used to send customized HTML code to the user's browser. We will write a CGI script that delivers stimuli in a randomly determined order to each participant. We'll build on the self-esteem survey that we developed in the previous chapter, but the general technique we'll develop can be applied in a variety of research contexts. Just as the order in which questionnaire items are presented can be randomized, we can randomize the stimuli when they're presented in other ways, such as with a series of images.

AN ILLUSTRATION

Copy the Perl code below to a blank document in your text editor. Save the file as randesteem1.pl in the cgi-bin directory on your server.

randesteem1.pl

```
#!C:/perl/bin/perl.exe
use CGI;
$query = new CGI;

$v01= "I feel that I'm a person of worth, at least
    on an equal plane with others.";
$v02= "I feel that I have a number of good qualities.
    ";
$v03= "All in all, I am inclined to feel that I am a
    failure.";
$v04= "I am able to do things as well as most other
    people.";
$v05= "I feel I do not have much to be proud of.";

print $query->header;
print $query->start_html(-title=>'Self-Esteem Test');

print "<FONT FACE = 'arial' SIZE = '2'>";
print "<B>This page is designed to assess your self-
    esteem.</B><BR> <BR>
Please answer the following questions. Once you have
    answered each question,
click the button labeled <I> calculate my score.</I>
    The web page will then calculate
```

```
your self-esteem score, and tell you more about how
    you compare to others.<BR><BR>";

print "<FORM ACTION = '/cgi-bin/self-esteem4.pl'
    METHOD = 'post'>";

@varlist = ("v01", "v02", "v03", "v04", "v05");

srand;
@new = ();
while (@varlist){
push(@new, splice(@varlist, rand @varlist,1));
}
@varlist= @new;

for($i = 0; $i <= 4; ++$i){
$question= $varlist[$i];
print " $$question <BR>";
print"<I>Strongly Disagree </I>
<INPUT TYPE = 'radio' NAME = $varlist[$i] VALUE = '1'>
<INPUT TYPE = 'radio' NAME = $varlist[$i] VALUE = '2'>
<INPUT TYPE = 'radio' NAME = $varlist[$i] VALUE = '3'>
<INPUT TYPE = 'radio' NAME = $varlist[$i] VALUE = '4'>
<INPUT TYPE = 'radio' NAME = $varlist[$i] VALUE = '5'>
<I>Strongly Agree</I><BR><BR><BR>";
}

print "<INPUT TYPE = 'submit' VALUE = 'Calculate my
    score'>";
print "</FORM></FONT>";
print $query->end_html;
```

Open your browser and go to the URL for this script. Recall that, because this script is a CGI script, it is located in the **cgi-bin** directory of your server. Notice that, unlike our previous examples, we're not searching for an HTML file (a file with an .htm extension). Instead, we're directly loading a CGI script.

Experiment with the program by "reloading" or "refreshing" the page in your browser. Each time you reload the page, you should see a new ordering of the five self-esteem questions. Don't submit any answers yet; we have yet to create the CGI script that will process the data.

FOR–NEXT LOOPS

Before we dissect the code of randesteem1.pl, I want to digress a moment to discuss for–next loops—another useful tool and one that will be used in many of the examples in the rest of this book. As we saw in the foreach example in Chapter 6, **loops** are coding instructions that perform the same task over and over again.

A for–next loop instructs the server to perform the same series of tasks a specified number of times (a number specified by the programmer). One of the important features of the for–next loop is that it uses an **index** variable, which monitors the number of times the server has passed through the loop.

It is necessary to understand and master for–next loops if you're going to do any complex programming, so let's begin with a discussion of a simple for–next loop. Enter the following script into a blank document and save it as fornextexample1.pl in your server's cgi-bin folder. After doing so, run the program in your browser (i.e., enter the full URL for the script—including the cgi-bin folder because this file is located inside the cgi-bin folder—into your browser address bar). On my server, the appropriate URL is http://www.web-research-design.net/cgi-bin/fornextexample1.pl.

fornextexample1.pl

```
#!C:/perl/bin/perl.exe
use CGI;
$query = new CGI;

print $query->header;
print $query->start_html(-title=>'For-Next Loop
    Example');

for($i = 0; $i <= 10; ++$i){
print "The index value is currently equal to $i.
    <BR><BR>";
}

print $query->end_html;
```

When you run this program, you should see the output illustrated in Figure 7.1.

Let's dissect the code and see how this loop works. As you can see from the output, the for–next loop is executing the print command within braces repeatedly. The number of times it executes that command is given in the

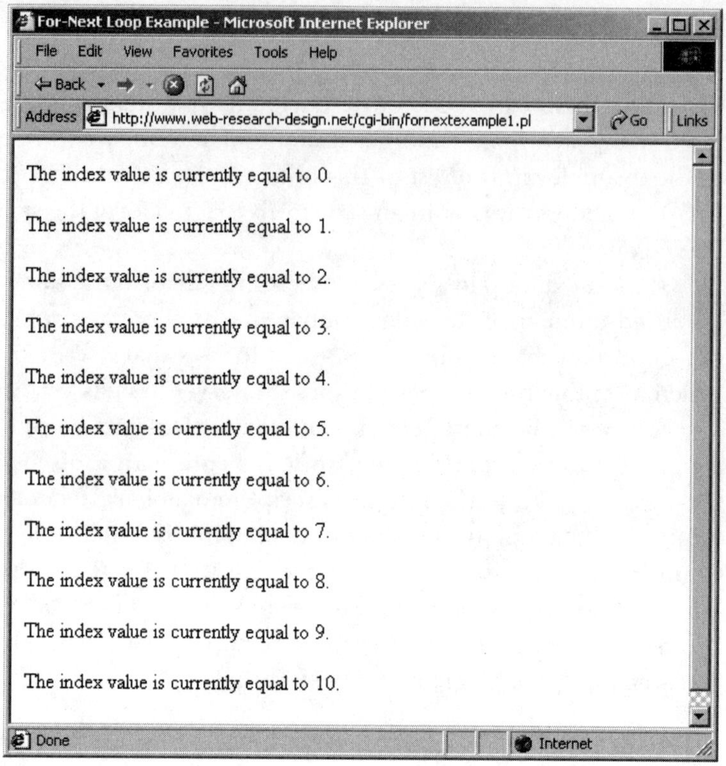

FIGURE 7.1. An illustration of looping operations and the role of the index value within the loop.

first line of the for-next command. The first part, $i = 0, tells the server *to begin* the loop by letting $i, the index variable, equal zero. The third part, ++$i, tells the server *to increment* the value of $i by 1 each time it finishes cycling through the commands in braces. (This is a Perl shorthand way of accomplishing $i = $i + 1.) The second part, $i <= 10, tells the server *to stop* cycling through the commands when $i is greater than 10. As long as $i is less than or equal to 10, the loop will continue. When $i equals 11, the server stops cycling through the loop.

In this example we begin the loop by letting $i equal 0. Next, the server executes the print command within braces (i.e., print "The index value is currently equal to $i.

"). Because $i currently equals

0, the user sees the following message, "The index value is currently equal to 0." Once the command has been executed, the server increments the value of $i by 1, making $i equal 1 (i.e., 0 + 1 = 1). Because $i is less than 11, the server returns to the beginning of the loop. The server again executes the command within braces. However, because $i now equals 1, the user sees the following message, "The index value is currently equal to 1." Once the server has finished executing this command, it increments $i by 1, so that it now equals 2 (i.e., 1 + 1 = 2). Because $i is still less than or equal to 11, the server returns to the beginning of the loop.

This process continues until $i equals 11. Notice that the last time through the loop, $i equals 10. The server then increments $i by 1, making $i equal 11. When it checks to see whether $i is equal to or less than 10, it discovers that $i is now greater than 10. As a consequence, the server quits executing the commands in braces and moves on to the next part of the program (in this case, the `print $query->end_html` command).

For–next loops are valuable because they allow you to execute repetitive commands easily. They are also helpful because the index value, $i, can be used in a variety of clever ways. One of those clever ways will be particularly useful to us; consider the following code:

fornextexample2.pl

```
#!C:/perl/bin/perl.exe
use CGI;
$query = new CGI;

print $query->header;
print $query->start_html(-title=>'Self-Esteem Test');
@names= ("Bumpy Molasses", "Spappy McNivens", "Winslow
    Pentiballo");

print "The first name is $names[0].<BR>";
print "The second name is $names[1].<BR>";
print "The third name is $names[2].<BR><BR><BR>";

for($i = 0; $i <= 2; ++$i){
print "The index value is currently equal to
    $i.<BR>";
print "The name corresponding to this index value is
    $names[$i].<BR><BR>";
}

print $query->end_html;
```

Copy this code to a blank document and save it as fornextexample2.pl in your server's cgi-bin directory. Open the program in your browser. When you run the program, you should see the output illustrated in Figure 7.2.

In this example we have created an **array** called @names that contains the names of three individuals. An array is a variable in Perl that contains multiple values or elements (see Chapter 5 for a more detailed discussion). Conveniently, we can refer to any element of this array by specifying its numerical index within the array by placing that number within brackets. For example, we can refer to element #1 of the array as $names[1]. It is important to note that *Perl begins counting with zero*, not one. Thus, in the three-element array discussed previously (i.e., @names), what we would normally consider to be the first element of the array is indexed numerically as the 0th element; the third element is indexed as the 2nd. This is easy to forget and cam be confusing, so, if a program involving arrays isn't working in the way you expect it to, check the indexing of the elements in your arrays.

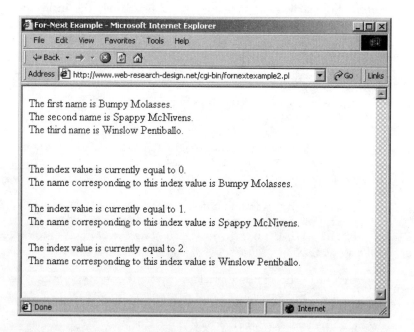

FIGURE 7.2. An example of how the index value can be used within a loop to refer to specific elements of an array.

> ### Note.
> When we are referring to *all* of the elements of an array (i.e., the array itself), we preface it with an ampersand (e.g., @names). When we are referring to a specific element in that array, we preface it with a dollar sign (e.g., $names[2]). Any one element of an array is a single value (scalar) and single values are referenced with dollar signs.

We can use the index number, $i, within a loop to reference a specific element in an array. In this example, the loop executes the commands within braces three times. The first time through, $i equals 0, and the server prints the 0th element of the array @names: "Bumpy Molasses." The second time through the loop, $i equals 1, and the server prints the 1st element of the array: "Spappy McNivens." The third time through, $i equals 2 and the server prints the 2nd element of the array: "Winslow Pentiballo." After its third time through, the server increments $i by 1, making $i equal to 3. Because 3 is greater than 2, the server exits the loop and moves to the next section of the programming code.

BREAKING DOWN THE CODE

Now that we have a better understanding of how for–next loops work, let's return to our randomization example, randesteem1.pl. The program begins with the same three lines we always begin our CGI scripts with. The first new aspect of the code is as follows:

```
$v01= "I feel that I'm a person of worth, at least
    on an equal plane with others.";
$v02= "I feel that I have a number of good
    qualities.";
$v03= "All in all, I am inclined to feel that I am a
    failure.";
$v04= "I am able to do things as well as most other
    people.";
$v05= "I feel I do not have much to be proud of.";
```

We're creating five local variables (i.e., $v01, $v02, . . . $v05) that contain the content of the five self-esteem items. Because the items are alphanumeric pieces of information, rather than numeric information per se, we treat them as *strings* and enclose the items in double quotes.

The next set of commands (e.g., print $query->header) should be familiar to you by now. We're instructing the CGI program to send a set of HTML codes to the user's browser. In particular, it will send it a set of codes that will print the instructions to the self-esteem questionnaire. Notice that these are the same instructions we used in the last chapter; however, in that chapter, the page was created from an HTML file proper. Here, the page is being created *entirely* by the CGI script.

The next code segment is a bit complicated.

```
@varlist = ("v01", "v02", "v03", "v04", "v05");
srand;
@new = ();
while (@varlist){
push(@new, splice(@varlist, rand @varlist,1));
}
@varlist= @new;
```

This segment begins simply enough. The first command instructs the server to create a local array called @varlist that will contain the values v01, v02, . . . v05. The next lines of code are responsible for taking this variable and randomly shuffling the order of the contents.

srand sets a random number seed—a number needed for generating random sequences. Next, we create a new, and temporary, local array called @new. By setting @new to equal the empty parentheses, we're telling Perl to create an array, but not to insert any content within it. Next, we begin a loop using the while command. The while command represents yet another kind of loop, with it we're going to randomly run through the contents of @varlist, one at a time, and push the contents into the array @new. Once each element of @varlist has been duplicated in this new array, the while loop ends. Finally, we copy over the old contents of @varlist by replacing them with the contents of @new—the new set of randomly shuffled elements.

It is not imperative that you understand the details of this code, so I won't elaborate on it in depth. It is important, however, that you understand its function. In short, this code takes the elements of the array @varlist and reorders them randomly. To use this code for your research purposes, all you'll need to do is insert the appropriate contents into @varlist. In this example, we're randomizing the order in which questionnaire items will be presented. Hence, the contents of @varlist are the symbolic names of the questions.

The next piece of code represents the real guts of the program. This segment employs a for–next loop to present each questionnaire item.

```
for($i = 0; $i <= 4; ++$i){
$question= $varlist[$i];
print " $$question <BR>";
print"<I>Strongly Disagree </I>
<INPUT TYPE = 'radio' NAME = $varlist[$i] VALUE = '1'>
<INPUT TYPE = 'radio' NAME = $varlist[$i] VALUE = '2'>
<INPUT TYPE = 'radio' NAME = $varlist[$i] VALUE = '3'>
<INPUT TYPE = 'radio' NAME = $varlist[$i] VALUE = '4'>
<INPUT TYPE = 'radio' NAME = $varlist[$i] VALUE = '5'>
<I>Strongly Agree</I><BR><BR><BR>";
}
```

Recall that we had previously randomized the order of elements within @varlist. For the purposes of discussion, let's assume that @varlist now contains the following ordering of elements: v03, v01, v05, v02, and v04.

The first thing the server does as it enters the for–next loop is to create an index variable, $i, and assign it the value zero. Next, it creates a local variable, $question, that will equal the *i*th element of the array @varlist. Because $i equals zero the first time through the loop, $question will be assigned the value "v03"—the 0th element of @varlist.

The next command is fairly subtle. In short, it instructs the server to print the value of $question. Importantly, however, it also instructs the server to print a dollar sign before it prints the value of $question. Because $question is equal to v03, the server interprets $$question as $v03. The server appends v03 to the dollar sign, and executes the following command:

```
print " $v03 <BR>";
```

Because $v03 has been assigned the text value of "All in all, I am inclined to feel that I am a failure," the program prints that questionnaire item to the user's browser.

The next few lines print the response options, as radio buttons, so that the user can click a response. The important thing to note here is what happens in the NAME attribute of the radio buttons. Because the order in which the questions are presented is random, we can't simply insert the names in the same way we did previously. Nonetheless, we still want to use the same names that we used before. For example, we want the response to question 3 to be named v03. To accomplish this, we take the ith element of @varlist and use that as the variable name: NAME = $varlist[$i]. The first time through the loop, when $i equals zero, the server will print question $v03 and the user's response will be named v03 (the 0th element of @varlist).

The second time through the loop, $i will be incremented by 1 and will equal 1. (The command, ++$i, is a shortcut for the command $i = $i + 1. Although this shortcut is less intuitive than $i = $i + 1, I have included it here because it is commonly used and you'll see it a lot in Perl examples you may find on the Internet.) The first 1st element of @varlist is v01. Therefore, the program appends v01 to a dollar sign, and prints out the contents of $v01. Next, it creates the radio button response options and names the response options v01. The program cycles through the loop, printing each questionnaire item and the corresponding radio buttons, until $i equals 6. At this point, the loop ends, and the server sends the browser the HTML code to produce the **Submit** button.

This loop probably seems fairly complex. I encourage you to study the commands in some depth, and experiment with alternative ways of creating the code (e.g., see what happens if you use the line print " $question
"; instead of print " $$question
";. Once you've experimented some with the code on your own, it should begin to feel more natural. Getting familiar with this code is important because we'll be using this looping trick often in the rest of this book in order to present stimuli. It is much easier to present the stimuli within the context of a loop as opposed to entering the appropriate code repeatedly for each stimulus you want to present.

PROCESSING AND SAVING RANDOMIZED DATA

Notice that from within randesteem1.pl we've instructed the server to run the self-esteem4.pl script when the **Submit** button is clicked. As you'll recall, this script, created in the last chapter, is designed to calculate the user's self-esteem score and save it to a data file called self-esteem.txt. You're probably wondering how the program is going to be able to calculate the subject's self-esteem score correctly given that the ordering of the questions will be different for each user. Recall, however, that we were able to name the response options appropriately. Although the user saw the questions in a randomized order, the NAME attribute for each response option retained the same names we used before (e.g., v01, v02).

To see for yourself that this is the case, open **randesteem1.pl** again in your browser window and right-click the white space in the window. This opens a new menu window; select the option **View Source**. You should be able to view the HTML code that the CGI script has sent to your browser window. Notice that the same response names we used before in our HTML file (e.g., v01, v02) are used here, but the items are listed in a different order than they were before. For example, the first item listed in Figure 7.3 is actually item v05, and the response to this item will be named v05 when it is sent to **self-esteem4.pl** in the CGI data packet for processing.

The fact that the NAME attributes for each item's response option still match the item name in the same way they did in the previous chapter is sig-

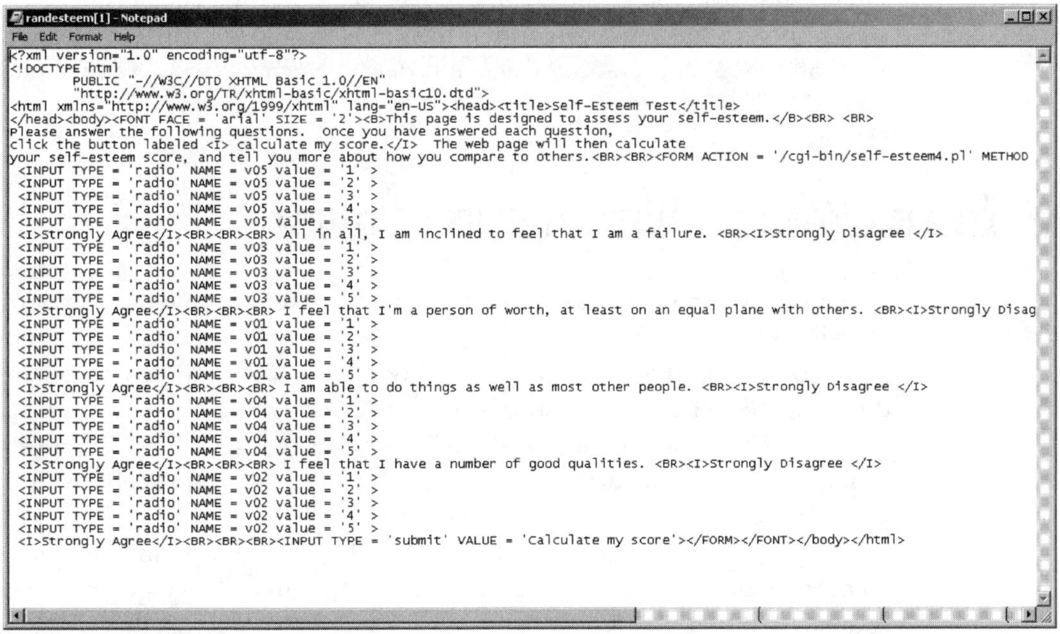


```
<?xml version="1.0" encoding="utf-8"?>
<!DOCTYPE html
        PUBLIC "-//W3C//DTD XHTML Basic 1.0//EN"
        "http://www.w3.org/TR/xhtml-basic/xhtml-basic10.dtd">
<html xmlns="http://www.w3.org/1999/xhtml" lang="en-US"><head><title>Self-Esteem Test</title>
</head><body><FONT FACE = 'arial' SIZE = '2'><B>This page is designed to assess your self-esteem.</B><BR> <BR>
Please answer the following questions.  Once you have answered each question,
click the button labeled <I> calculate my score.</I>  The web page will then calculate
your self-esteem score, and tell you more about how you compare to others.<BR><BR><FORM ACTION = '/cgi-bin/self-esteem4.pl' METHOD
 <INPUT TYPE = 'radio' NAME = v05 value = '1' >
 <INPUT TYPE = 'radio' NAME = v05 value = '2' >
 <INPUT TYPE = 'radio' NAME = v05 value = '3' >
 <INPUT TYPE = 'radio' NAME = v05 value = '4' >
 <INPUT TYPE = 'radio' NAME = v05 value = '5' >
 <I>Strongly Agree</I><BR><BR><BR> All in all, I am inclined to feel that I am a failure. <BR><I>Strongly Disagree </I>
 <INPUT TYPE = 'radio' NAME = v03 value = '1' >
 <INPUT TYPE = 'radio' NAME = v03 value = '2' >
 <INPUT TYPE = 'radio' NAME = v03 value = '3' >
 <INPUT TYPE = 'radio' NAME = v03 value = '4' >
 <INPUT TYPE = 'radio' NAME = v03 value = '5' >
 <I>Strongly Agree</I><BR><BR><BR> I feel that I'm a person of worth, at least on an equal plane with others. <BR><I>Strongly Disag
 <INPUT TYPE = 'radio' NAME = v01 value = '1' >
 <INPUT TYPE = 'radio' NAME = v01 value = '2' >
 <INPUT TYPE = 'radio' NAME = v01 value = '3' >
 <INPUT TYPE = 'radio' NAME = v01 value = '4' >
 <INPUT TYPE = 'radio' NAME = v01 value = '5' >
 <I>Strongly Agree</I><BR><BR><BR> I am able to do things as well as most other people. <BR><I>Strongly Disagree </I>
 <INPUT TYPE = 'radio' NAME = v04 value = '1' >
 <INPUT TYPE = 'radio' NAME = v04 value = '2' >
 <INPUT TYPE = 'radio' NAME = v04 value = '3' >
 <INPUT TYPE = 'radio' NAME = v04 value = '4' >
 <INPUT TYPE = 'radio' NAME = v04 value = '5' >
 <I>Strongly Agree</I><BR><BR><BR> I feel that I have a number of good qualities. <BR><I>Strongly Disagree </I>
 <INPUT TYPE = 'radio' NAME = v02 value = '1' >
 <INPUT TYPE = 'radio' NAME = v02 value = '2' >
 <INPUT TYPE = 'radio' NAME = v02 value = '3' >
 <INPUT TYPE = 'radio' NAME = v02 value = '4' >
 <INPUT TYPE = 'radio' NAME = v02 value = '5' >
 <I>Strongly Agree</I><BR><BR><BR><INPUT TYPE = 'submit' VALUE = 'Calculate my score'></FORM></FONT></body></html>
```

FIGURE 7.3. The HTML code that was generated by our **randesteem1.pl** Perl script.

nificant. When the self-esteem4.pl script is executed, it will be able to extract the correct information from the submitted data packet because the responses have been assigned the correct names.

You're probably also wondering how we're going to save the information to the data file in a standard way since the questions are appearing in a different order for each subject. Fortunately, when we wrote our self-esteem4.pl script to save the data, we used the following command:

```
print INFO "$v01, $v02, $v03, $v04, $v05,";
```

Thus, Perl will save the data in the same order for each participant (i.e., $v01 will be saved first, followed by $v02, and so on), regardless of the order in which the items were presented to our participant. To see this for yourself, I encourage you to experiment with randesteem1.pl some more. Specifically, note the order in which the questions are presented to you, and then record on a piece of paper the actual answers you gave to the questions. After you submit your data, open the self-esteem.txt data file. You should notice that your responses have been organized by variable name (i.e., $v01, $v02, $v03, $v04, and $v05) and not in the actual order in which you answered the questions.

ANOTHER EXAMPLE, WITH A SLIGHT TWIST

I want to work through another example in order to illustrate how randomly shuffling the elements of an array—in combination with the use of for–next loops—can be used to randomize a different kind of stimuli. Instead of randomizing the order of questionnaire items, let's randomize the order in which visual stimuli are presented. We'll use three images here. Also, instead of saving the data to a data file, we'll e-mail it to ourselves (to keep the example simple).

Copy the following code to a blank document and save it as randexample.pl in your cgi-bin directory. (Be sure to change the e-mail address in the FORM tag to your own. Also, don't forget to download the appropriate images to the images folder on your server [see Chapter 3]. If you don't have the images on your server, the images will not be displayed for your participants.)

randexample.pl

```perl
#!C:/perl/bin/perl.exe
use CGI;
$query = new CGI;

$v01= "/images/image1.jpg";
$v02= "/images/image2.jpg";
$v03= "/images/image3.jpg";

print $query->header;
print $query->start_html(-title=>'Mental Rotation');

print "<FONT FACE = 'arial' SIZE = '2'>";
print "<B>Image Rating Example.</B><BR> <BR>
Each image depicts two objects. In some cases, one
   object is a simple rotation of the other. In other
   cases, the two objects are not the same. For each
   image, decide whether the objects are the
   <I>same</I> (i.e., one is a simple rotation of the
   other) or whether they are <I>different</I>.
   <BR><BR>";

print "<FORM ACTION = 'mailto:fraley\@uic.edu' METHOD
   = 'post' ENCTYPE = 'text/plain'>";

@varlist = ("v01", "v02", "v03");

srand;
@new = ();
while (@varlist){
push(@new, splice(@varlist, rand @varlist,1));
}
@varlist= @new;

print "<CENTER>";

for($i = 0; $i <= 2; ++$i){
$image= $varlist[$i];
print "<IMG SRC=$$image><BR>";
print "<TABLE><TR><TD ALIGN='center'>
<I>Same</I><BR>
<INPUT TYPE = 'radio' NAME = $varlist[$i] VALUE = '1'>
</TD>";
print "<TD ALIGN='center'><I> Different</I><BR>
<INPUT TYPE = 'radio' NAME = $varlist[$i] VALUE = '2'>
</TD></TR></TABLE><BR>";
}
```

```
print "<INPUT TYPE = 'submit' VALUE = 'Submit my
   responses'>";
print "</FORM></FONT></CENTER>";
print $query->end_html;
```

> **Note.** In the code above, I used a backslash before the @ in my e-mail address: `fraley\@uic.edu`. Although you do not need to do this in a proper HTML document (i.e., one with an .htm or .html extension), when you're including this HTML command **within a CGI script** (i.e., in a file with the .pl extension), the server will process the @ symbol in a way other than its intended purpose here. Therefore, to instruct the server to interpret the @ symbol literally (i.e., as @), include the slash.

This demonstration employs images similar to those used by Shepard and Metzler (1971) in their classic research on mental imagery and rotation. The screen depicted in Figure 7.4 should be similar to the one you will see when you enter the appropriate URL in your browser.

Notice that this script has the same structure as the previous one. The only exceptions are as follows:

• We have three stimuli instead of five. As a consequence, @varlist only contains three elements, and the commands within our for–next loop will only be executed three times.

• The stimuli, instead of being questionnaire items, are images. We've assigned the URL for the images to separate variables (i.e., $v01, $v02, $v03), and have substituted the variable name into the HTML tag for displaying an image.

• When the program reaches the `$image= $varlist[$i]` command within the loop, it takes the *i*th element of @varlist and lets it equal $image. The first time through the loop, when $i equals 0, the program takes the 0th element of @varlist, v01, and assigns that to the variable $image. Thus, if we assume that we hadn't randomized @varlist and the 0th element was v01, $image would now equal v01. In the next line, `print "<IMG SRC=$$image><BR>"`, we place a dollar sign in front of $image, thereby tricking the program into seeing $v01 instead of just v01. Because the code will appropriately interpret $v01 as a representing a variable, it substitutes the contents of $v01, `/images/image1.jpg`, into the command. In other words, the program reads the line as if it said: `print "<IMG SRC = '/images/image1.jpg'><BR>"` instead of `print "<IMG SRC=$$image><BR>"`.

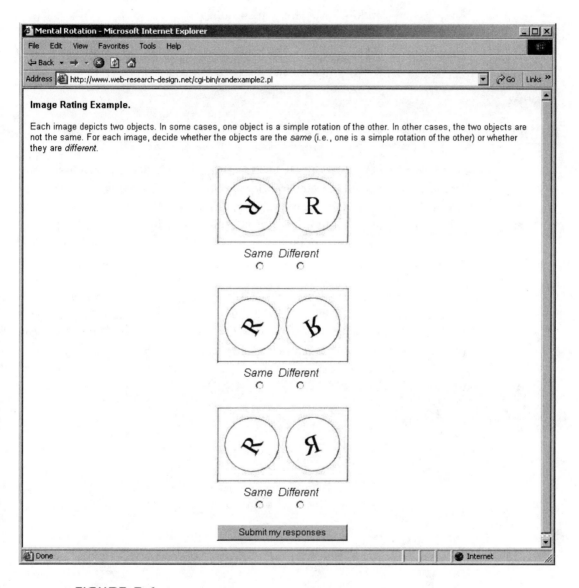

FIGURE 7.4. Images, like text, can be presented in a random order to each participant.

- Every time we click the refresh or reload button on our browser, we obtain a new random order for the stimuli.

> **Note.** Remember that, to use images as stimuli, those images need to be saved to the **images** folder within your **Public HTML** folder.

A FINAL EXAMPLE, WITH A BIGGER TWIST

There may be cases in which you want to present participants with, say, five items that have been selected randomly from a bank of, say, ten items. To accomplish this, you can use the same techniques that we've discussed before with a minor twist. Namely, instead of allowing the for–next loop to present *all* the available stimuli, we limit it so that it presents only a subset of those stimuli.

Let's return to the self-esteem example to illustrate. Let's assume that we had a data base of 10 possible self-esteem items, but we only wanted to present a random subset of 5 of those 10 items to the participant. Instead of setting the for–next loop to cycle through the loop commands 10 times, we can instruct it to cycle through 5 times. Here is some example code to experiment with. Copy the code and save it as **randesteem2.pl** to your server's **cgi-bin** directory.

randesteem2.pl

```
#!C:/perl/bin/perl.exe
use CGI;
$query = new CGI;

$v01= "I feel that I'm a person of worth, at least
    on an equal plane with others.";
$v02= "I feel that I have a number of good
    qualities.";
$v03= "All in all, I am inclined to feel that I am a
    failure.";
$v04= "I am able to do things as well as most other
    people.";
$v05= "I feel I do not have much to be proud of.";
$v06= "I take a positive attitude toward myself.";
$v07= "On the whole, I am satisfied with myself.";
$v08= "I wish I could have more respect for myself.";
$v09= "I certainly feel useless at times.";
```

```perl
$v10= "At times I think I am no good at all.";

print $query->header;
print $query->start_html(-title=>'Self-Esteem Test');

print "<FONT FACE = 'arial' SIZE = '2'>";
print "<B>This page is designed to assess your self-
    esteem.</B><BR> <BR>";

print "<FORM ACTION = 'mailto:fraley\@uic.edu' METHOD
    = 'post' ENCTYPE = 'text/plain'> ";

@varlist = ("v01", "v02", "v03", "v04", "v05", "v06",
    "v07", "v08", "v09", "v10");

srand;
@new = ();
while (@varlist){
push(@new, splice(@varlist, rand @varlist,1));
}
@varlist= @new;

for($i = 0; $i <= 4; ++$i){
$question= $varlist[$i];
print " $$question <BR>";
print"<I>Strongly Disagree </I>
<INPUT TYPE = 'radio' NAME = $varlist[$i] VALUE = '1'>
<INPUT TYPE = 'radio' NAME = $varlist[$i] VALUE = '2'>
<INPUT TYPE = 'radio' NAME = $varlist[$i] VALUE = '3'>
<INPUT TYPE = 'radio' NAME = $varlist[$i] VALUE = '4'>
<INPUT TYPE = 'radio' NAME = $varlist[$i] VALUE = '5'>
<I>Strongly Agree</I><BR><BR><BR>";
}

print "<INPUT TYPE = 'submit' VALUE = 'Submit my
    scores'>";
print "<BR><BR>Thank you.<BR></FORM></FONT>";
print $query->end_html;
```

For simplicity, I have constructed this example so that the data will be e-mailed to the researcher, rather than stored by the server. However, I encourage you to write a CGI script that will process and store the data. The "challenge" is that the form will send different variables each time since the variables are being randomly selected. This can be handled fairly easily, but will require some clever code manipulation on your part. (See the web page for this book, http://www.web-research-design.net/, for one simple solution.)

SUMMARY

The objective of this chapter was to demonstrate a general technique for randomizing the presentation order of stimuli. Although we focused mainly on randomizing questionnaire items, it should be clear that we can use this technique to randomize other types of things we might want to present to people over the Internet.

In this chapter we learned the following:

1.   It is possible to use a **for–next** loop to execute repetitive commands. For example, if we're using the same response scale for a large number of questionnaire items, we can simply stick the INPUT tags within the loop, and separately print each questionnaire item as the program passes through each cycle of the loop.

2.   The for–next loop is a useful type of loop which uses an **index** number to track the number of times the program has cycled through the loop. This index number, often (but not necessarily) designated as $i, can be used to identify or refer to specific elements of an array.

3.   The elements of an array can be randomly shuffled. As a consequence, you can easily randomize the order of stimuli. Once the order has been randomized, you can present your stimuli, one at a time, controlled by the for–next loop.

4.   If you want to select only a handful of stimuli from a larger bank of stimuli, you can randomly shuffle the elements of an array and then limit the for–next loop so that it presents fewer stimuli than the total number available.

Here is a review of the Perl codes that were introduced in this chapter.

Perl commands	Function	Example
`for(begin, end, increment){}`	A for–next loop executes a set of commands a specified number of times. The loop uses an index variable which is incremented each time the commands within braces are executed. *begin* specifies the value of the index when the loop begins; *end* specifies the value of the index that causes the loop to end, and increment specifies the manner in which the index value is incremented with each pass of the loop. `++$i` is a common command used to increment the loop by 1 unit each time through.	`for($i = 0; $i <= 10;` `++$i){` `print "The index value is` `currently equal to $i.` `  ";` `}` (These commands create a for–next loop that begins with $i equal to 0. Each time through the loop, $i is incremented by 1. The commands within braces are executed each time until the value of $i is greater than 10.)
`@array = ("a", "b", "c");` `srand;` `@new = ();` `while (@array){` `push(@new,` `splice(@array, rand` `@array,1));` `}` `@array = @new;`	This block of commands can be used to randomly shuffle the elements in a previously defined array. This is a useful way to randomize the presentation order of a set of stimuli.	`@varlist= ("v01", "v02",` `"v03", "v04", "v05");` `srand;` `@new = ();` `while (@varlist){` `push(@new, splice(@varlist,` `rand @varlist,1));` `}` `@varlist= @new;` (This set of commands randomly shuffles the elements of the @varlist array: v01, v02, v03, v04, v05.)

Chapter 8

Random Assignment to Conditions

One of the most important aspects of research design in the behavioral sciences is random assignment of participants to conditions. The use of random assignment helps to ensure that there are no systematic factors—other than the experimental manipulation—that might explain participants' responses. In this chapter I will show you how to randomly assign people to conditions by building on the randomization techniques we discussed in the previous chapter.

AN EXAMPLE

Let's assume we are interested in studying the factors that underlie judgments people make about the qualifications of job applicants. More specifically, let's assume that we want to know how much the sex of the applicant matters in the way the applicant is evaluated. To investigate this issue, we can construct a simple one-factor, between-subjects experiment in which participants read a short description of a person's qualifications for a job and rate the quality of the applicant. In one condition, participants are told that the person to be evaluated is a man. In the other condition, participants are told that the person to be evaluated is a woman.

Let's begin by creating two HTML web pages that contain the qualifications of a hypothetical candidate for an imaginary academic position in cognitive psychology. On one page, the applicant will be described as a man. On the other, the applicant will be described as a woman. Here is the HTML code for both pages. (I've kept the material as short as possible in order to conserve space.) Copy the first page to a blank document and save it as **randassign-a.htm** in your **Public HTML** folder. Copy the second page to a blank document and save it as **randassign-b.htm** in your **Public HTML** folder. Be sure to replace my e-mail address with yours in the code below.

randassign-a.htm

```
<HTML>
<TITLE>Job Study</TITLE>
<FORM ACTION = 'mailto:fraley@uic.edu' METHOD = 'post'
   ENCTYPE ='text/plain'>
<B>Please read the following description of a job
   candidate for a tenure-track cognitive position in
   your department. After reading this description,
   please indicate how qualified you believe this
   person to be for the job.</B>
<BR><BR>
<CENTER>Applicant 3<BR></CENTER>
This applicant received her PhD one year ago from the
   University of Illinois at Chicago. Her research is
   concerned with understanding the cognitive
   mechanisms underlying individual differences in
   working memory capacity. She has published four
   articles in peer-reviewed journals, on two of which
   she was first author.
<BR><BR><BR>
How qualified do you think this individual is for the
   job position?<BR>
<I>Not at all qualified </I>
<INPUT TYPE='radio' NAME = 'v01' VALUE = '1'>
<INPUT TYPE='radio' NAME = 'v01' VALUE = '2'>
<INPUT TYPE='radio' NAME = 'v01' VALUE = '3'>
<INPUT TYPE='radio' NAME = 'v01' VALUE = '4'>
<INPUT TYPE='radio' NAME = 'v01' VALUE = '5'>
<I> Strongly qualified </I><BR><BR>
```

```
<INPUT TYPE='hidden' NAME = 'condition' VALUE =
   'female'>
<INPUT TYPE = 'submit' VALUE ='Submit my
   evaluation'></FORM>
</HTML>
```

randassign-b.htm

```
<HTML>
<TITLE>Job Study</TITLE>
<FORM ACTION = 'mailto:fraley@uic.edu' METHOD = 'post'
   ENCTYPE ='text/plain'>
<B>Please read the following description of a job
   candidate for a tenure-track cognitive position in
   your department. After reading this description,
   please indicate how qualified you believe this
   person to be for the job.</B><BR><BR>
<CENTER>Applicant 3<BR></CENTER>
This applicant received his PhD one year ago from the
   University of Illinois at Chicago. His research is
   concerned with understanding the cognitive
   mechanisms underlying individual differences in
   working memory capacity. He has published four
   articles in peer-reviewed journals, on two of which
   he was first author.<BR><BR><BR>
How qualified do you think this individual is for the
   job position?<BR>
<I>Not at all qualified </I>
<INPUT TYPE = 'radio' NAME = 'v01' VALUE = '1'>
<INPUT TYPE = 'radio' NAME = 'v01' VALUE = '2'>
<INPUT TYPE = 'radio' NAME = 'v01' VALUE = '3'>
<INPUT TYPE = 'radio' NAME = 'v01' VALUE = '4'>
<INPUT TYPE = 'radio' NAME = 'v01' VALUE = '5'>
<I> Strongly qualified </I><BR><BR>
<INPUT TYPE = 'hidden' NAME = 'condition' VALUE =
   'male'>
<INPUT TYPE = 'submit' VALUE ='Submit my
   evaluation'></FORM>
</HTML>
```

Notice that the applicant description for the two candidates is identical. The only thing we've varied is whether the applicant is described as a female (randassign-a.htm) or male (randassign-b.htm).

Our next task is to randomly assign our participant to see one (and only one) of these two web pages. Copy the following script to a blank document and save it as randassign.pl in your server's cgi-bin folder.

randassign.pl

```
#!C:/perl/bin/perl.exe
use CGI;
$query = new CGI;

@filelist = ("randassign-a.htm", "randassign-b.htm");
srand;
@new = ();
while (@filelist){
push(@new, splice(@filelist, rand @filelist,1));
}
@filelist= @new:

$selectedfile= $filelist[0];
print $query->redirect("/$selectedfile");
```

The purpose of this CGI script is to randomly assign the participant to one of the two conditions. To accomplish this task, notice that we've used the same randomization techniques discussed in the previous chapter. Specifically, we created an array that contains the file name corresponding to each condition of our experiment (i.e., randassign-a.htm and randassign-b.htm). Next, we randomly shuffled the order of those files. Then we selected the 0th element of @filelist. Since @filelist has been randomly shuffled, we expect the 0th element to be randassign-a.htm 50% of the time. Finally, using the $query-> redirect() command, we instruct the server to go to the randomly selected web page.

Let's test this script. Type the URL for the CGI script, randassign.pl, into your browser address bar. Because there are no HTML codes contained in the CGI script, you shouldn't see anything at first. The script, however, will quickly redirect you to a new page, either randassign-a.htm or randassign-b.htm. Run the randassign.pl script a few times. (You'll probably need to type in the URL again since the script has taken you to a new page.) You should find that, on average, you'll be redirected to the male page 50% of the time. Figure 8.1 illustrates an example of what the randassign-a.htm page looks like in the browser.

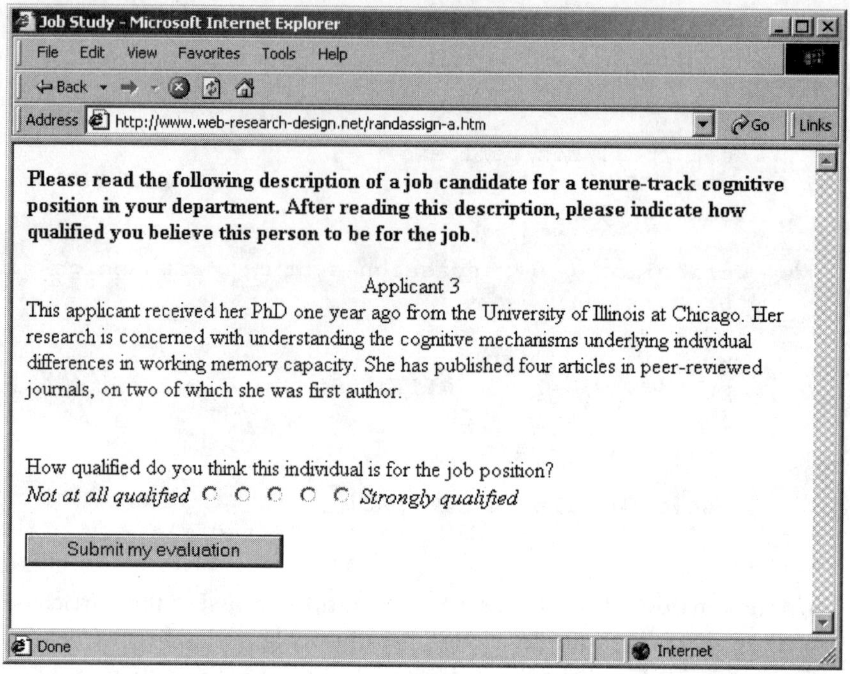

FIGURE 8.1. This page represents one condition of a between-subjects design involving two conditions.

Note. For the purposes of illustration, we've named the two files **randassign-a** and **randassign-b**. This naming convention, however, implies that there is more than one page associated with this experiment. If your subjects notice this aspect of the file name, they might get curious and begin entering similar filenames to see what happens. This, of course, will interfere with your experiment. It is ideal to generate filenames that do not appear to be obvious variants of the same theme (e.g., **a183721.htm**). Avoid filenames such as **condition1.htm** or **femaletarget.htm**. Later in the chapter I'll show you an approach to random assignment that eliminates the problem completely.

Notice that we've placed a hidden value within each of the two web pages corresponding to the condition. This value will be e-mailed to us, along with the user's rating. If we did not include this hidden value, we would not know whether the user's rating corresponded to the male or female target.

ANOTHER WAY TO IMPLEMENT RANDOM ASSIGNMENT

The method discussed above is a relatively simple way to randomly assign people to conditions. Moreover, as you might imagine, the technique can be extended to situations in which you have more than two conditions. If we were conducting a 3 × 3 between-subjects experiment, for example, we would have 9 conditions total, and we would extend the @filelist array to contain the HTML pages corresponding to all 9 of those conditions.

There is another way to implement random assignment that can be advantageous, especially when the stimuli are relatively simple. Specifically, we use the CGI script to present the HTML code rather than having it redirect the user to one of many different pages. One of the advantages of this technique is that the user will not see a filename that might clue him or her into the fact that different conditions exist.

Copy the following code into a blank document and save it as randassign2.pl in your server's cgi-bin directory.

randassign2.pl

```perl
#!C:/perl/bin/perl.exe
use CGI;
$query = new CGI;

$conda= "This applicant received her PhD one year ago
    from the University of Illinois at Chicago. Her
    research is concerned with understanding the
    cognitive mechanisms underlying individual
    differences in working memory capacity. She has
    published four articles in peer-reviewed journals,
    on two of which she was first author.";

$condb= "This applicant received his PhD one year ago
    from the University of Illinois at Chicago. His
    research is concerned with understanding the
    cognitive mechanisms underlying individual
    differences in working memory capacity. He has
    published four articles in peer-reviewed journals,
    on two of which he was first author.";

@condlist = ("$conda", "$condb");
srand;
@new = ();
while (@condlist){
```

```
push(@new, splice(@condlist, rand @condlist,1));
}
@condlist= @new;
$selectedcond= $condlist[0];

print $query->header;
print $query->start_html(-title=>'Job Study');
print "<FORM ACTION = 'mailto:fraley\@uic.edu' METHOD
    = 'post' ENCTYPE ='text/plain'>";
print "<B>Please read the following description of a
    job candidate for a tenure-track cognitive position
    in your department. After reading this description,
    please indicate how qualified you believe this
    person to be for the job.</B><BR><BR>
<CENTER>Applicant 3<BR></CENTER>";

print "$selectedcond";

print "<BR><BR><BR>
How qualified do you think this individual is for the
    job position?<BR>
<I>Not at all qualified </I>
<INPUT TYPE='radio' NAME = 'v01' VALUE = '1'>
<INPUT TYPE='radio' NAME = 'v01' VALUE = '2'>
<INPUT TYPE='radio' NAME = 'v01' VALUE = '3'>
<INPUT TYPE='radio' NAME = 'v01' VALUE = '4'>
<INPUT TYPE='radio' NAME = 'v01' VALUE = '5'>
<I> Strongly qualified </I><BR><BR>";

if($condlist[0] eq "$condb"){
print "<INPUT TYPE='hidden' NAME = 'condition' VALUE=
    'male'>";
}

if($condlist[0] eq "$conda"){
print "<INPUT TYPE='hidden' NAME = 'condition' VALUE=
    'female'>";
}

print "<INPUT TYPE = 'submit' VALUE ='Submit my
    evaluation'></FORM>";
print "</FORM>";
print $query->end_html;
```

Now, type the URL for **randassign2.pl** into your browser's address bar. You should see a page that looks identical to one of the two pages we saw previously. Click on **Refresh** or **Reload** a couple of times. You should note that the sex of the participant is male about half of the time.

If you study the code you'll see that we've employed a combination of randomly shuffling elements and simple variable substitution to pull this off. In short, we defined two local variables, $conda and $condb, each of which contains the appropriate text for one of the two levels of the manipulation. We placed these variables within an array called @condlist, randomly shuffled the array, and then selected the 0th element from the new array. We then used this element, either $conda or $condb, in the HTML code that was printed to the user's browser. The only other piece of code worth noting here is the hidden value. If the 0th element of @condlist is equal to $condb, then a hidden value is sent with the HTML code that codes the condition as "male." If the 0th element of @condlist is $conda, then a hidden value is sent equal to "female." If we do not send a hidden value along with the response, we will not know which condition the user was assigned to when the data are submitted. If we include this hidden value, we will receive an e-mail that tells us both what condition the user had been assigned to and his or her rating.

MANIPULATING VARIABLES WITHIN-SUBJECTS

In the previous chapter, we illustrated the technique of random shuffling arrays to randomize the order in which stimuli are presented. It should be clear that the same technique can be used to manipulate a variable within-subjects. If the "things" being shuffled are stimuli from different levels of a within-subjects manipulation, then the same randomization techniques can be applied to randomize the order of these stimuli. In this case, however, we'll often want the stimuli to appear on separate web pages rather than all appearing on the same page. In the next chapter, we'll discuss one way to use multiple pages in a research context.

SUMMARY

In this chapter we have covered two techniques for randomly assigning people to different experimental conditions. One simple way to implement random assignment is to create separate web pages or HTML documents for each experimental condition and have a Perl script redirect the user to one of those pages. Another way is to include the varied material (e.g., a narrative description of a job candidate) as local variables within a Perl script and have the script randomly determine which material will be presented. The second way is preferable because (1) it only requires one file and (2) your user cannot use the name of the web page to deduce the fact that other conditions exist.

Here is a review of the Perl codes that were introduced in this chapter.

Perl commands	Function	Example
`print $query-> redirect("URL");`	The redirect command automatically redirects the user to a different web page or CGI script.	`print $query-> redirect("http://www. google.com");`

Chapter 9

Using Multiple Web Pages in Research

Carrying Responses Forward from One Page to the Next

The examples we have focused on up to this point presented *all* the stimuli on a single web page. There may be situations, however, in which you want to present stimuli on separate pages. If you're presenting images as stimuli, for example, you might want to present one image per page so that the user's browser doesn't become overwhelmed by having to download a large number of image files at once. Moreover, if you're manipulating a variable within-subjects, you may not want the stimuli for each condition to appear on the same page.

Unfortunately, there is a problem in working with multiple pages. When the user submits data to the server from a web page, the server processes the information and immediately "dissolves" its relationship with the user. Thus, if the user submits new data from a separate page, the server does not recognize the fact that the same user is sending new information. The transactions between the user's computer and the server are said to be *stateless*. In other words, once the server passes information to the user (via submitting data from a form), it has no memory for the transaction. If the user were to answer questions from another web page of the study and submit those, the server has no way to know that it is the user submitting new data from a different page of the same study.

There are, of course, a number of ways around this problem, and we'll focus on one useful method in the present chapter. Specifically, we will use **hidden tags** to pass information back and forth between the server and the user's browser. To get a sense of how this might work, imagine that we're having our participants answer five questions, one per page. Once the user submits his or her response from the first page, the CGI script extracts the response from the form, encodes it as a hidden value, and prints that response, as well as the new question, as part of the second HTML page. Thus, when the user submits his or her response to the second question, that response *as well as the response to the first question* (which is encoded as a hidden value), is sent to the server. By extending this process across multiple pages, it is possible to keep a record of a user's previous responses despite the fact that the server per se experiences complete amnesia each time it interacts with the user.

AN EXAMPLE

To illustrate this process, let's return to the self-esteem example. Instead of presenting the five self-esteem questions on a single page, let's present one item at a time, each on a different page. Copy the following two scripts and save them as multiform1.pl and multiform2.pl, respectively, in the cgi-bin directory of your server.

multiform1.pl

```
#!C:/perl/bin/perl.exe
use CGI;
$query = new CGI;

print $query->header;
print $query->start_html(-title=>'Self-Esteem Test');
```

```
print "<FONT FACE = 'arial' SIZE = '2'>";
print "<FORM ACTION = '/cgi-bin/multiform2.pl' METHOD
   = 'post'>";
print "Welcome to the self-esteem survey. Please click
   the button to begin.<BR>";
print "<INPUT TYPE = 'hidden' NAME = pass VALUE = 0>";
print "<INPUT TYPE = 'submit' VALUE = 'Next'>";
print "</FORM></FONT>";

print $query->end_html;
```

multiform2.pl

```
#!C:/perl/bin/perl.exe
use CGI;
$query = new CGI;

$v01= $query->param('v01');
$v02= $query->param('v02');
$v03= $query->param('v03');
$v04= $query->param('v04');
$v05= $query->param('v05');
$pass= $query->param('pass');

$q01= "I feel that I'm a person of worth, at least
   on an equal plane with others.";
$q02= "I feel that I have a number of good
   qualities.";
$q03= "All in all, I am inclined to feel that I am a
   failure.";
$q04= "I am able to do things as well as most other
   people.";
$q05= "I feel I do not have much to be proud of.";

@varlist= ("v01", "v02", "v03", "v04", "v05");
@qlist= ("q01", "q02", "q03", "q04", "q05");

print $query->header;
print $query->start_html(-title=>'Self-Esteem Test');

print "<FONT FACE = 'arial' SIZE = '2'>";
print "<FORM ACTION = '/cgi-bin/multiform2.pl' METHOD
   = 'post'> ";

if($pass <= 4){
$question= $qlist[$pass];
```

```
print " $$question <BR>";
print"<I>Strongly Disagree </I>
<INPUT TYPE = 'radio' NAME = $varlist[$pass] VALUE = '1'>
<INPUT TYPE = 'radio' NAME = $varlist[$pass] VALUE = '2'>
<INPUT TYPE = 'radio' NAME = $varlist[$pass] VALUE = '3'>
<INPUT TYPE = 'radio' NAME = $varlist[$pass] VALUE = '4'>
<INPUT TYPE = 'radio' NAME = $varlist[$pass] VALUE = '5'>
<I>Strongly Agree</I><BR><BR><BR>";
    for($i = 0; $i <= 4; ++$i)
    {
    $variable= $varlist[$i];
    print "<INPUT TYPE = 'hidden' NAME = $variable
    VALUE = $$variable > ";
    }
$pass = $pass + 1;
print "<INPUT TYPE = 'hidden' NAME = pass VALUE =
    $pass > ";
print "<INPUT TYPE = 'submit' VALUE = 'Next'>";
print "</FORM></FONT>";
}

else{
print "</FORM>";
print "<FORM ACTION = '/cgi-bin/self-esteem.pl' METHOD
    = 'post'> ";
print "You've answered all the questions. Click the
    button
below to determine your self-esteem score.<BR><BR>";
    for($i = 0; $i <= 4; ++$i)
    {
    $variable= $varlist[$i];
    print "<INPUT TYPE = 'hidden' NAME = $variable
    VALUE = $$variable > ";
    }
    print "<INPUT TYPE = 'submit' VALUE = 'Calculate
    my score'>";
    }

print $query->end_html;
```

Open your browser and enter the URL for multiform1.pl into the address bar. The first thing you should see is a simple page that says, "Welcome to the self-esteem survey. Please click the button to begin," and a **Submit** button labeled Next. Press the **Submit** button. The next page should contain a single questionnaire item, a response scale, and a **Submit** button labeled Next. Once you respond to the item and click the Next button, a new page will load with a different self-esteem item. After you've answered each of the five questions, you will see a page stating that you've answered all the questions. The new **Submit** button will be labeled, **Calculate my score**.

Let's break down the code and see how it works. All of the code should be familiar to you by now; there are no new Perl commands in this program. What is new, however, is the specific way we've used the commands to present the items across pages. Let's focus on some of these tricks.

The first script, multiform1.pl, is a simple introductory script that welcomes the user to the study. It does, however, serve a function more important than this. Specifically, when the **Submit** button is pressed, a hidden variable named "pass" whose value is 0 will be submitted to the server. As will be explained in more depth below, this hidden value will be used to tell the next script, multiform2.pl, that the user has not answered any questions up to this point.

Now let's study the next script—multiform2.pl. The first thing to notice is that there are commands for two HTML forms embedded in this script. The first form is used whenever the number of questions the subject has answered is less than 5, or, more precisely, when the value of $pass is less than or equal to 4. When the subject has answered all five questions, a new form is constructed. We have used the if–else command to determine which of these two HTML forms will be transmitted to the user's browser.

For now, let's examine the HTML form that is created when the research participant has not answered all the questions. The first thing to note is that the ACTION attribute for the FORM tag contains the URL for the script in question. In other words, when the user clicks the **Submit** button, he or she activates multiform2.pl again or (else) self-esteem.pl at the end. Because the server–browser relationship is stateless, the server won't think this is odd. It simply runs the script again as if nothing unusual has taken place. Fortunately, the script is written in a manner that causes it to behave differently depending on the kind of information that has been submitted to it. Each time it is activated, the script will be working with different information, so it will not always behave in the same way.

The first few lines of the script are designed to read in CGI data that have been submitted to the server. Notice that the script is reading in values for questions 1 through 5 (i.e., v01 through v05) even though the user hasn't answered any questions yet. This is okay and will not cause the program to run incorrectly. The script will read in any values that exist and assign them to the appropriate local variables. If the variables were not sent in the CGI packet, the script will simply ignore the commands.

One of the variables the script reads is "pass." Specifically, the script looks for a variable called "pass" in the CGI data packet and, if it exists, assigns its value to the local variable $pass. Recall that we submitted a variable called "pass" as a hidden value when we triggered multiform2.pl by pressing the **Submit** button in multiform1.pl. Thus, the first time multiform2.pl is activated, it reads in a hidden variable called "pass" and assigns its value (which happens to be 0) to a local variable called $pass. We will use this variable to denote how many questions that user has answered—how many times the user has passed through this script.

The next significant section of code is contained in the if($pass <= 4) condition. These commands are executed whenever the value of $pass is less than or equal to 4. The first time the script is activated, the user has not answered any questions; therefore, the value of $pass is 0. Because 0 is less than 4, the commands within braces are executed.

What do these commands do? These commands print a questionnaire item for the user, as well as a response scale and a **Submit** button labeled **Next.** Because $pass equals 0, the 0th element of @qlist is the item that is presented to the user. The response value will be given the name corresponding to the 0th element of @varlist. The general strategy that we're using here for looping through items is the same strategy that we used in Chapter 7.

When the user presses the **Submit** button, we not only want to pass along the user's rating for the item, but we also want to pass along information about how many questions the user has answered thus far. To do this, we simply add 1 to the value of $pass and then create a hidden variable tag that contains the updated value of $pass. Now, after answering the first question, the user will pass along his or her rating as well as a hidden variable called "pass" which will equal 1.

Notice that we also included a simple for-next loop in order to pass along as hidden values information about each response (i.e., v01, v02, v03, v04, and v05). This allows us to pass along the responses as we collect them and, thereby, overcome the inherent statelessness of the exchange between the server and the user. The importance of this step will become more clear below.

Let's assume the user responds the first time through by clicking the third radio button, thereby setting the value of v01 to 3. Once the user enters a response and clicks **Next,** the same script that was just run is run again. This time, however, there are more data in the CGI data packet than there were previously. This time, there is a value of 3 corresponding to v01, which was passed forward in a hidden tag. Therefore, a local variable named $v01 is created and assigned the value of 3. We also passed forward responses to the other items (e.g., v02, v03) as hidden values, but, because the user hasn't responded to these items yet, the hidden tags contain no information. As a consequence, the corresponding local variables that are created for each of these variables (e.g., $v02, $v03) are empty. Also, and importantly, the value of "pass" in the data packet is 1, so the script creates a local variable called $pass and sets it equal to 1.

After creating these local variables, the script presents the user with the 2nd questionnaire item. (This is represented as the 1st element of @qlist.) Let's assume the user enters a value of 5 for this question and clicks the **Submit** button. Now, a data packet is sent to the server that contains *three* important pieces of information: v01 = 3, v02 = 5, and pass = 2. The first piece of information, v01 = 3, is encoded as a hidden value corresponding to a response from a previous trial, the second is an explicit response from the user to the questionnaire item he or she just saw and is also passed along as a hidden value.

Notice that this cycle of transactions continues to take place between the server and the user's browser until the fifth question had been administered (i.e., until $pass equals 5). When the response to that final question has been submitted, the value of "pass" that the server submits is 5. Thus, when the script is activated again, the server skips past the `if($pass <= 4)` condition since it is no longer true and executes instead the commands within the `else` braces.

```
else{
  print "</FORM>";
  print "<FORM ACTION = '/cgi-bin/self-esteem.pl'
    METHOD = 'post'> ";
  print "You've answered all the questions. Click the
    button below to determine your self-esteem
    score.<BR><BR>";
    for($i = 0; $i <= 4; ++$i)
    {
```

```
        $variable= $varlist[$i];
        print "<INPUT TYPE = 'hidden' NAME = $variable
        VALUE = $$variable > ";
        }

    print "<INPUT TYPE = 'submit' VALUE = 'Calculate my
      score'>";
    }
```

These commands do several things. First, the FORM tag that was previously open is closed: `print "</FORM>"`. Second, a new FORM tag is opened: `print "<FORM ACTION = '/cgi-bin/self-esteem.pl' METHOD = 'post'>"`. This tag instructs the server to activate the self-esteem.pl script when the **Submit** button is clicked. Recall from previous chapters that the self-esteem.pl script is responsible for computing a person's self-esteem score and saving the data. Third, the script prints new information to the user. Specifically, it tells the user that he or she has answered each question, and that he or she should click the **Submit** button to have his or her self-esteem score computed. Finally, with the help of a for–next loop, the server prints all of the self-esteem responses as hidden values. These data are now passed to the self-esteem.pl script when the user presses the **Submit** button.

RANDOMIZING TRIALS ACROSS MULTIPLE WEB PAGES

The example we just explored presented the self-esteem questions in the same order for each user. I constructed the program in this manner in order to present the technique of carrying information from one page to the next as simply as possible. In advanced research applications, however, you will want to randomize the order of the stimuli and present them on separate pages.

To do so, we can simply combine the techniques we discussed previously in the context of randomization with those discussed in this chapter. The following example will randomize the order of the questions, as well as present each question on a separate page. We'll use two scripts to accomplish this. The first script will be responsible for generating the random order of the questions. The second will be responsible for presenting the questions in that random order.

Copy the following code to a blank document and save it as randmultiform1.pl in your server's cgi-bin folder.

randmultiform1.pl

```perl
#!C:/perl/bin/perl.exe
use CGI;
$query = new CGI;

@varlist= ("01", "02", "03", "04", "05");
srand;
@new = ();
while (@varlist){
push(@new, splice(@varlist, rand @varlist,1));
}
@varlist= @new;

print $query->header;
print $query->start_html(-title=>'Self-Esteem Test');
print "<FONT FACE = 'arial' SIZE = '2'>";
print "<FORM ACTION = '/cgi-bin/randmultiform2.pl'
   METHOD = 'post'> ";
print $query->hidden('varlist',@varlist);
print "Welcome to the self-etseem survey. Please click
   the button to begin.<BR><BR>";
print "<INPUT TYPE = 'hidden' NAME = pass VALUE = 0
   > ";
print "<INPUT TYPE = 'submit' VALUE = 'Begin'>";
print "</FORM></FONT>";

print $query->end_html;
```

Also copy the following code to a blank document and save it as randmultiform2.pl in your server's cgi-bin folder.

randmultiform2.pl

```perl
#!C:/perl/bin/perl.exe
use CGI;
$query = new CGI;

@varlist= $query->param('varlist');
$v01= $query->param('v01');
$v02= $query->param('v02');
$v03= $query->param('v03');
$v04= $query->param('v04');
$v05= $query->param('v05');
$pass= $query->param('pass');
```

```perl
$q01= "I feel that I'm a person of worth, at least
    on an equal plane with others.";
$q02= "I feel that I have a number of good
    qualities.";
$q03= "All in all, I am inclined to feel that I am a
    failure.";
$q04= "I am able to do things as well as most other
    people.";
$q05= "I feel I do not have much to be proud of.";

print $query->header;
print $query->start_html(-title=>'Self-Esteem Test');

print "<FONT FACE = 'arial' SIZE = '2'>";
print "<FORM ACTION = '/cgi-bin/randmultiform2.pl'
    METHOD = 'post'> ";

if($pass <= 4){
$question= $varlist[$pass];
$question= "q" . $question;
$variable= $varlist[$pass];
$variable= "v" . $variable;
print " $$question <BR>";
print"<I>Strongly Disagree </I>
<INPUT TYPE = 'radio' NAME = $variable VALUE = '1'>
<INPUT TYPE = 'radio' NAME = $variable VALUE = '2'>
<INPUT TYPE = 'radio' NAME = $variable VALUE = '3'>
<INPUT TYPE = 'radio' NAME = $variable VALUE = '4'>
<INPUT TYPE = 'radio' NAME = $variable VALUE = '5'>
<I>Strongly Agree</I><BR><BR><BR>";
    for($i = 0; $i <= 4; ++$i)
    {
    $variable= $varlist[$i];
    $variable= "v" . $variable;
    print "<INPUT TYPE = 'hidden' NAME = $variable
    VALUE = $$variable > ";
    }
$pass = $pass + 1;
print $query->hidden('varlist',@varlist);
print "<INPUT TYPE = 'hidden' NAME = pass VALUE =
    $pass > ";
print "<INPUT TYPE = 'submit' VALUE = 'Next'>";
print "</FORM></FONT>";
}
```

```
else{
  print "</FORM>";
  print "<FORM ACTION = '/cgi-bin/self-esteem.pl'
    METHOD = 'post'> ";
  print "You've answered all the questions. Click the
    button below to determine your self-esteem
    score.<BR><BR>";
    for($i = 0; $i <= 4; ++$i)
    {
    $variable= $varlist[$i];
    $variable= "v" . $variable;
    print "<INPUT TYPE = 'hidden' NAME = $variable
    VALUE = $$variable > ";
    }
  print "<INPUT TYPE = 'submit' VALUE = 'Calculate my
    score'>";
  }

print $query->end_html;
```

The first script performs a few important tasks. First, it randomizes the sequence in which the self-esteem questions will be presented. Notice that it uses the same random shuffling technique we've used before. Second, the page serves as an introductory page, briefly explaining to the participant what the web page is all about. Third, when the **Submit** button is pressed, the code will activate a new script, randmulitform2.pl, and pass to that script two hidden variables. One of those hidden variables is the "pass" variable that we discussed in the previous section. This variable indicates the number of times the user has passed through randmultiform2.pl and is set to 0 at the beginning of the study. The second hidden variable contains the array @varlist which represents the randomized order for presenting the stimuli.

> **Note.** One cannot simply use the standard HTML expression for a hidden tag (e.g., `<INPUT TYPE = 'hidden' NAME = 'varlist' VALUE = @varlist>`) when the information is an array rather than a single value. However, it is possible to pass an array in a hidden tag by using the following command:
> `print $query->hidden('varlist',@varlist);`

The second script, randmultiform2.pl, works in the same way as the multiform2.pl script discussed earlier in this chapter. There are, however, a few new tricks in here. First, this script, in addition to trying to read in v01, v02, . . . v05 from the submitted data packet, is reading in @varlist—the array containing the randomized order in which the questions are to be presented. Recall that this information has been passed to the script from randmultiform1.pl via a hidden tag. Second, this script passes along @varlist as a hidden tag so that the next time the script is called, will have access to those values. This process allows the user and the server to transcend the inherent statelessness of their interactions. Third, this script employs a highly useful append function in Perl. Consider the following lines of code:

```
$question= "q" . $question;
$variable= "v" . $variable;
```

The use of the period instructs Perl to piece these two fragments together. If the value of $question was 01, by appending that to "q," we end up with q01.

> **Note.** To **append** two strings in Perl, we can insert a period between the two fragments. For example, if we wanted to create the string "coffeecup" from the fragments "coffee" and "cup," we would use the following command: $newstring = "coffee" . "cup";. You can use the period to append literal strings, as just illustrated, or variables. For example, if we had two variables, $x and $y, we could append them with the following command: $newvariable = $x . $y;. If $x was equal to "coffee" and $y was equal to "cup," this command would produce the same output as the one shown above.

In order to better understand some of the things these scripts are doing, I encourage you to dissect them on your own. Include commands to print the contents of certain variables and arrays so you can see exactly what they look like, and what their values are at different points in the process. Change things around a bit and see how that affects the operation of the scripts. Finally, try to customize these scripts with questionnaire items of your own. (You will, of course, need to modify the **self-esteem.pl** program if you experiment too much. The easiest way to experiment with these programs safely is to change the final form so that, instead of passing the data packet to **self-esteem.pl**, it passes it to you via e-mail.)

USING IMAGE MAPS TO ADVANCE FROM ONE PAGE TO THE NEXT

One of the limitations of the technique we've just discussed is that each page requires two mouse clicks for the user, one for rating the item and one for submitting the response and advancing to the next page. One way to minimize the number of clicks is to use an *image map* for both the response scale and the **Submit** button (see Chapter 4). When users click on an image map, the browser records the exact pixel that was clicked and automatically submits whatever data was collected.

To see an image map in action, run the randmultiform3.pl script on the web page for this book (http://www.web-research-design.net/cgi-bin/randmultiform3.pl). After a brief introduction page, which randomizes the order of the stimuli behind the scene, you will be taken to a new page where you will be asked to rate a self-esteem item by clicking somewhere on the rating scale that corresponds to your response. An example screenshot is presented in Figure 9.1.

Notice that there is not a separate "submit" button on this web page. As soon as you click somewhere along the scale, you will be taken to the next page. By using the image-based rating scale as an image map, we are able to use one click to both record the response and advance to the next page or question.

The three scripts below are used to implement this study. Copy the following scripts to blank documents and save them as randmultiform3.pl, randmultiform4.pl, and self-esteem-coord.pl, respectively, in your server's cgi-bin folder.

randmultiform3.pl

```
#!C:/perl/bin/perl.exe
use CGI;
$query = new CGI;

@varlist= ("01", "02", "03", "04", "05");
srand;
@new = ();
while (@varlist){
push(@new, splice(@varlist, rand @varlist,1));
}
@varlist= @new;
```

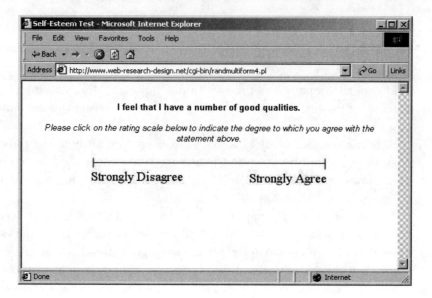

FIGURE 9.1. Here an image map collects the response, submits the data, and advances the user to the next page or item.

```
print $query->header;
print $query->start_html(-title=>'Self-Esteem Test');

print "<FONT FACE = 'arial' SIZE = '2'>";
print "<FORM ACTION = '/cgi-bin/randmultiform4.pl'
   METHOD = 'post'> ";
print $query->hidden('varlist',@varlist);
print "Welcome to the self-esteem survey. Please click
   the button to begin.<BR><BR>";
print "<INPUT TYPE = 'hidden' NAME = 'pass' VALUE =
   '0'> ";
print "<INPUT TYPE = 'submit' VALUE = 'Begin'>";
print "</FORM></FONT>";

print $query->end_html;
```

randmultiform4.pl

```
#!C:/perl/bin/perl.exe
use CGI;
$query = new CGI;
```

```
@varlist= $query->param('varlist');
$v01x= $query->param('v01.x');
$v02x= $query->param('v02.x');
$v03x= $query->param('v03.x');
$v04x= $query->param('v04.x');
$v05x= $query->param('v05.x');
$pass= $query->param('pass');

$q01= "I feel that I'm a person of worth, at least
   on an equal plane with others.";
$q02= "I feel that I have a number of good
   qualities.";
$q03= "All in all, I am inclined to feel that I am a
   failure.";
$q04= "I am able to do things as well as most other
   people.";
$q05= "I feel I do not have much to be proud of.";

print $query->header;
print $query->start_html(-title=>'Self-Esteem Test');

print "<FONT FACE = 'arial' SIZE = '2'>";
print "<FORM ACTION = '/cgi-bin/randmultiform4.pl'
   METHOD = 'post'> ";

for($i = 0; $i <= 4; ++$i)
    {
    $variable= $varlist[$i];
    $hiddenvariablename= "v" . $variable . ".x";
    $variable= "v" . $variable . "x";
    print $query->hidden($hiddenvariablename,$$variable);
    }

if($pass <= 4){
    $question= $varlist[$pass];
    $question= "q" . $question;
    $variable= $varlist[$pass];
    $variable= "v" . $variable;
    print "<CENTER><BR>";

print "<B> $$question </B><BR><BR>";
print " <I>Please click on the rating scale below to
   indicate the degree to which you agree with the
   statement above.</I> <BR><BR>";
```

```perl
print"<INPUT TYPE='image' SRC='/images/scale.jpg' NAME
    = $variable ></CENTER><BR>";
$pass = $pass + 1;
print $query->hidden('varlist',@varlist);
print "<INPUT TYPE = 'hidden' NAME = pass VALUE =
    $pass > ";
print "</FORM></FONT>";
}
```

self-esteem-coord.pl

```perl
#!C:/perl/bin/perl.exe
use CGI;
$query = new CGI;
$v01x= $query->param('v01.x');
$v02x= $query->param('v02.x');
$v03x= $query->param('v03.x');
$v04x= $query->param('v04.x');
$v05x= $query->param('v05.x');

$esteem = ($v01x + $v02x + (364 - $v03x) + $v04x +
    (364 - $v05x) ) /5;
$esteem2 = sprintf("%.2f", $esteem);

($sec,$min,$hour,$mday,$mon,$year,$wday,$yday,$isdst) =
    localtime(time);
$ip= $query->remote_addr();
open(INFO, ">>$ENV{'DOCUMENT_ROOT'}/www/data/self-
    esteem-coord.txt");
 print INFO "$mon/$mday/$year\, ";
 print INFO "$hour:$min:$sec\, ";
 print INFO "$ip, ";
 print INFO "$v01x, $v02x, $v03x, $v04x, $v05x,";
 print INFO "$esteem2, ";
 print INFO "endline \n";
close (INFO);

$sum= 0;
$n= 0;

open(INFO, "$ENV{'DOCUMENT_ROOT'}/www/data/self-esteem-
    coord.txt");
@data = <INFO>;
close(INFO);

foreach $key (@data)
```

```
{
($adate,$atime,$aip,$av01,$av02,$av03,$av04,$av05,
   $aesteem2,$aendline)=split(/,/,$key);
$sum= $sum + $aesteem2;
$n= $n + 1;
}

$esteemmean= $sum/$n;
$esteemmean = sprintf("%.2f", $esteemmean);

print $query->header;
print $query->start_html(-title=>'Thank You');
print "<FONT FACE = 'arial' SIZE = '2'><B>Self-Esteem
   Results Page</B><BR><BR>
Your self-esteem score is $esteem2, on a scale
   ranging from 1 to 364.<BR><BR>
The average self-esteem score for people who have
   taken this survey is $esteemmean.<BR><BR>
To date, $n people have taken this survey.
</FONT>";
print $query->end_html;
```

To run this online study, open your browser and enter the URL for randmultiform3.pl into the address bar. This first script, randmultiform3.pl, like the randmultiform1.pl script we discussed previously, is responsible for welcoming the participant and randomizing the order of the stimuli. It is identical to randmultiform1.pl with one exception: after randomizing the stimuli, it runs randmultiform4.pl, which is responsible for presenting the actual questionnaire items in a manner that allows the user's previous responses to be carried forward from one page to the next. Instead of collecting the ratings via a radio-button based rating scale, however, this script uses an image map.

When an image map is clicked by a user, the *x* and *y* coordinates of the pixel that was clicked are passed to the server, along with any other form information that was collected (e.g., hidden values, additional form responses). As discussed in Chapter 4, the browser appends ".x" and ".y" to the name of the image map in order to separate these distinct pieces of information. Thus, if a user clicks on an image map named v01, two new variables, v01.x and v01.y, which represent the *x* and y coordinates of the pixel that was clicked, will be passed to the server. As a consequence, we need to make sure that the script is able to account for the fact that browsers automatically append ".x" and ".y" to the name of input from image maps.

The first thing we need to do to account for this is to modify the lines of the code in which the program reads the $query or CGI data. For example, we have changed the line $v01= $query->param('v01') to read $v01x= $query->param('v01.x'). By doing so, we are reading in information from a CGI variable called v01.x and assigning it to a local variable called $v01x. The second thing we have done is adjust the way the *x*-coordinate of the click for each item is passed from one page to the next via hidden value tags.

```
$variable= $varlist[$i];
$hiddenvariablename= "v" . $variable . ".x";
$variable= "v" . $variable . "x";
print $query->hidden($hiddenvariablename,$$variable);
```

In this code we've created a new variable, $hiddenvariablename, that will represent the name of the *x*-coordinate for a specific trial. Thus, if we are passing the *x*-coordinate recorded for variable 2 (i.e., v02), we create the appropriate variable name by appending "02" to "v" and appending ".x" to that string. This allows us to create a name, v02.x, for the *x*-coordinate that we can pass to the next page via a hidden value tag. Importantly, we must pass the information from an image map along in the same way that the browser would do so. In other words, we're *mimicking* the labeling conventions of the browser by appending a ".x" to the name of the image map value that we're passing along.

Notice that we're not changing the value for the variable; we're only changing the name that the value is given. By naming the variable in this manner, we can successfully pass the previous responses forward from one page to the next because, each time the script is activated, it will search the $query data for v01.x, v02.x, v03.x, v04.x, and v05.x.

The **self-esteem-coord.pl** script is designed to save the data, process the user's data and respond with his or her average self-esteem score, as well as the average self-esteem score of the rest of the participants. This script is similar to the **self-esteem3.pl** script discussed in Chapter 6. The major difference is that it accounts for the fact that the responses to the self-esteem items will not range between 1 and 5. Because this particular rating scale is 363 pixels wide, the *x*-axis pixel location can range anywhere between 0 and 363. As a consequence, we need to reverse key two of the items appropriately, and explain to the user the possible range of scores.

It should be noted that we only used information about the *x*-coordinate in this example. There may situations in which information about the *y*-coordinate of the click is desirable as well. The procedures that would be used to obtain and pass along information about the *y*-coordinate are identical to those used to pass along information about the *x*-coordinate.

SUMMARY

There are many research situations in which it may be desirable to present stimuli on multiple pages as opposed to a single page. Unfortunately, the stateless nature of the interaction between the server and a user does not automatically provide for information collected from one page to be carried forward to the next. In order to overcome this limitation, the user's responses can be carried along in the form of hidden tags. By constructing a CGI script that systematically reads in each response from the data packet and prints the responses obtained thus far as hidden tags, you can transcend statelessness.

Here is a review of the Perl commands that were introduced in this chapter.

Perl commands	Function	Example
`print $query->hidden('arrayname',@array);`	To pass along hidden arrays, use this command, where arrayname represents the variable/array name (similar to the NAME attribute of an HTML hidden tag) and @array represents the array you want to pass along. In general, it is useful to use this format for passing hidden variables via CGI scripts rather than the HTML format. Although the HTML format will generally work, this format is more robust.	`print $query->hidden ('varlist',@varlist);` (In this example, the array, @varlist, is passed along in a hidden tag called varlist.)
`$newvariable= $variable1 . $variable2;`	The use of a period allows you to *append* two variables together.	`$newvariable= "v" . "at";` (This example creates a new local variable, $newvariable, that equals "vat.") `$newvariable= "c" . $y;` (This example creates a new local variable, $newvariable, that equals "cat"; $y is equal to "at.")

Chapter 10

Using Conditional Branching Structures

An Example of "Skip Patterns" in Survey Research

There are many situations in behavioral research where the kinds of stimuli to be presented in one trial will depend on the way the participant has responded in previous trials. A common example is the use of *skip patterns* in survey research. If a participant indicates that he or she is married, you may want to probe the participant in more depth about the marriage. If the participant is not married, you will need him or her to skip ahead to the next set of relevant questions. In a paper-and-pencil context, skipping ahead can distract or confuse participants. Participants might misunderstand the instructions, or they might skip too far ahead in the survey. When questions are administered online, however, we can have the CGI script do the skipping automatically.

In this chapter I'll show you how to implement conditional branching structures. I'll highlight the case of "skip patterns" in surveys, but of course, these general techniques can be used to implement conditional branching structures other research contexts, as well.

Let's work with a simple, five-question survey. Here is what it would look like on paper:

1. Are you married?
   ☐ Yes
   ☐ No (If "no," skip ahead to question 5.)

2. How long have you been married?
   _____ years

3. Do you have any children with your current spouse?
   ☐ Yes
   ☐ No (If "no," skip ahead to question 5.)

4. How many children do you have?

   _____

5. Are you male or female?
   ☐ Male
   ☐ Female

Notice that the various "pathways" through the survey have a clear logical structure. For example, if the answer to question 1 is "yes," the respondent moves on to question 2. If the respondent answers "no," the respondent moves ahead to question 5.

Before constructing a CGI program to implement these branching patterns, it would be useful to create a map of the logical structure entailed by the questions. Figure 10.1 shows the logical structure of the survey. Notice that if you know which question a respondent is currently answering, you can determine exactly where he or she needs to go next, depending on the answer provided. Our goal is to implement this logical structure in our CGI program.

Copy the following script into a blank document and save it as **skippatterns.pl** in your server's **cgi-bin** directory.

skippatterns.pl

```
#!C:/perl/bin/perl.exe
use CGI;
$query = new CGI;
```

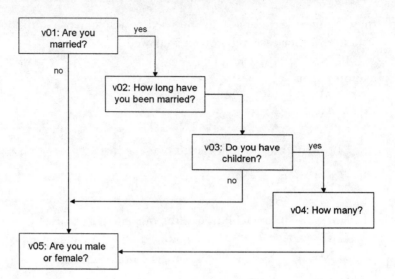

FIGURE 10.1. This diagram shows the branching structure implied by our questionnaire. We want to implement this logical structure within our Perl script.

```
$v01=  $query->param('v01');
$v02=  $query->param('v02');
$v03=  $query->param('v03');
$v04=  $query->param('v04');
$v05=  $query->param('v05');
$lastposition=  $query->param('lastposition');

#------------------------
if($lastposition  ==  0){
    $thisposition=1;
}
#------------------------
if($lastposition==1){
  if($v01==1){
    $thisposition=  2;
    }
  else{
    $thisposition=5;
    }
}
#------------------------
if($lastposition==2){
```

```
        $thisposition=3;
}
#----------------------
if($lastposition==3){
  if($v03==1){
    $thisposition= 4;
    }
  else{
    $thisposition=5;
    }
}
#----------------------
if($lastposition==4){
    $thisposition=5;
}
#----------------------
if($lastposition==5){
    $thisposition=6;
}
#----------------------

print $query->header;
print $query->start_html(-title=>'Branching Pattern
   Demonstration');
print "<FONT FACE = 'arial' SIZE = '2'>";

if ($thisposition != 6){

    print "<FORM ACTION = '/cgi-bin/skippatterns.pl'
    METHOD = 'post'> ";

    if($thisposition ==1){
      print "Are you married? <BR>";
      print "<INPUT TYPE = 'radio' NAME = 'v01' value
         = 0> No <BR>";
      print "<INPUT TYPE = 'radio' NAME = 'v01' value
         = 1> Yes <BR>";
      $lastposition=1;
    }

    if($thisposition==2){
      print "How many years have you been married?
         <BR>";
      print "<INPUT TYPE = 'textbox' NAME = 'v02'
        MAXLENGTH=2 SIZE=2> years<BR>";
    $lastposition=2;
    }
```

```
if($thisposition==3){
   print "Do you have any children with your
      current spouse? <BR>";
   print "<INPUT TYPE = 'radio' NAME = 'v03' value
      = 0> No <BR>";
   print "<INPUT TYPE = 'radio' NAME = 'v03' value
      = 1> Yes <BR>";
$lastposition=3;
}

if($thisposition==4){
   print "How many children do you have? <BR>";
   print "<INPUT TYPE = 'textbox' NAME = 'v04'
      MAXLENGTH=2 SIZE=2><BR>";
$lastposition=4;
}

if($thisposition==5){
   print "Are you male or female? <BR>";
   print "<INPUT TYPE = 'radio' NAME = 'v05' value
      = 0> Male <BR>";
   print "<INPUT TYPE = 'radio' NAME = 'v05' value
      = 1> Female <BR>";
$lastposition=5;
}

print "<INPUT TYPE = 'hidden' NAME = 'v01' VALUE
   = $v01>";
print "<INPUT TYPE = 'hidden' NAME = 'v02' VALUE
   = $v02>";
print "<INPUT TYPE = 'hidden' NAME = 'v03' VALUE
   = $v03>";
print "<INPUT TYPE = 'hidden' NAME = 'v04' VALUE
   = $v04>";
print "<INPUT TYPE = 'hidden' NAME = 'v05' VALUE
   = $v05>";
print "<INPUT TYPE = 'hidden' NAME =
   'lastposition' VALUE = $lastposition>";
print "<INPUT TYPE = 'submit' VALUE = 'Next
   Question'>";
print "</FORM>";
}

#-------------------------------

else{
```

```
open(INFO,
   ">>$ENV{'DOCUMENT_ROOT'}/www/data/skipdemo.txt");
print INFO "$v01, $v02, $v03, $v04, $v05\n";
close(INFO);
print "Thank you for your participation. Your data
   have been saved.<BR>";
print "</FORM>";
}

print $query->end_html;
```

Run this program and see what it does.

We're not introducing any new Perl commands in this script, so I'll just broadly summarize the logic of the program and how it works. We begin by reading in variables from $query. However, the first time the script is run, no data packet is submitted. As a consequence, the various local variables, such as $v01 and $lastposition are empty.

The next section of the code contains a series of if–then conditions that allow the server to determine where the user is in the map. We're going to use the variables **$lastposition** and **$thisposition** to represent where we came from and where we need to be, respectively.

Note. The **#** sign can be used in a Perl script as a comment. In other words, if you want to partition your code or insert comments in your code that you don't want Perl to interpret as real commands, insert a pound sign at the beginning of the document line or to the left of where you want the comment to start. In the code above I've used the pound sign along with a series of dashes to help separate the different parts of the code. When Perl reaches a pound sign, it ignores everything to the right of the sign to the end of the line. You can take advantage of this to create comments to yourself within the code or, in the case of trying to debug your program, to "comment out" specific lines of code to see if those lines are the source of a problem. By commenting out a line of code you instruct the server to ignore it temporarily rather than your having to delete it and retype it later.

The first time through the script, $lastposition is empty (which is analogous to containing a value of zero). Thus, the first condition is satisfied: "$lastposition equals zero." As a consequence, a local variable called $thisposition is created and set equal to 1. This represents the fact that the user is coming from question 0 (he or she hasn't had any questions yet) and, therefore, needs to be presented with question 1.

After testing the next conditions, the server reaches a condition that is true: "$thisposition equals 1." Therefore, the server executes the commands within braces. These commands print the first question to the user's browser, as well as the corresponding response options. Finally, the server displays a **Submit** button that will cause the user to move on to the next question whenever he or she is ready. It is noteworthy that, after this condition is met, the server updates the value of $lastposition to 1, and places this value in a hidden tag. Thus, when the user clicks the **Submit** button, he or she is submitting not only a response to the first question, but also information about where he or she is in the logical map.

Once the **Submit** button is pressed, the script reloads (the ACTION attribute of the FORM tag refers to skippatterns.pl), reads the information in the current CGI data packet, and assigns the new values to local variables based on that information. Specifically, this second time through, $v01 now contains a numeric value and the value of $lastposition is 1. When the server now sorts through the various conditions, it finds that the condition "$lastposition equals 1" is satisfied. This tells the server that the user just completed the first question. In order to determine where to go next, the server examines the response to the first question. If $v01 is equal to 1, the server sets $thisposition to 2; if not, the server sets $thisposition to 5. Recall that we're using the variable $thisposition to code for which question the server should ask in the current round.

If $thisposition was set to 2, then the server proceeds to ask the second question. If $thisposition was set to 5, then the server asks the fifth question. After the fifth question, $thisposition is assigned a value of 6. The commands we just studied were executed only if the value of $thisposition was not equal to (less than) 6. Now that it is equal to 6, the server saves the data and thanks the user for his or her participation.

SUMMARY

It is possible to use CGI scripting to create a unique pathway for the visitor to travel. By passing the user's current location in the branching map via hidden tags, and using the appropriate if–then conditions, it is possible to save your user the hassle of having to skip over irrelevant questions manually.

Chapter 11

Advanced Feedback

Summarizing Data with Bar Graphs and Two-Dimensional Plots

In Chapter 6 we discussed ways to provide subjects with feedback about their responses. Specifically, I described how to average the responses within a sample so users can see how their scores compare to those of others. We also discussed the use of if–then conditions to further customize feedback.

So far, the feedback we have provided to users has been text-based, not graphical. There may be contexts, however, in which you want to create graphical feedback for your users. There are at least two ways to implement graphing techniques in CGI. The first method would be to download and import a special program called GD.pm (http://stein.cshl.org/www/software/GD). GD.pm is a group of Perl operations written by Lincoln Stein that is designed to interface with Thomas Boutell's GD program (http://www.boutell.com.gd). GD and GD.pm can be used to create customized, on-the-fly graphics with Perl. Unfortunately, the documentation for installing and using the needed programs is sparse and assumes a high degree of technical expertise.

The second method involves combining simple, premade images

arramged creatively in HTML tables. For our purposes, this method has many advantages over GD.pm. First, it doesn't require any new knowledge on our part. Everything we need to know to pull this off has been covered in previous chapters. Second, using HTML tables to format and organize simple images doesn't require much computation on the server's part. Finally, we don't need to install any new software to use this method.

In this chapter we'll discuss this simple approach in order to create two kinds of graphs that are commonly used in behavioral research: bar graphs and two-dimensional coordinate plots.

BAR GRAPHS

Consider the following image:

This image is so small that you probably cannot even see it. The image file, bargray.jpg (which can be downloaded from this book's website: http://www.web-research-design.net/), contains only a single gray pixel.

In HTML code, we can insert this image using the IMG tag: `<IMG SRC='/images/bargray.jpg'>`.

Recall that we can adjust the height and width of the displayed image in the IMG tag by manipulating the WIDTH and HEIGHT attributes: `<IMG SRC='/images/bargray.jpg' WIDTH='80' HEIGHT='20'>`. This code would produce a bar similar to the one illustrated in Figure 11.1.

Notice that we've taken an image of pixel size 1 × 1 and stretched it so it is displayed at a pixel size of 80 × 20. By adjusting these dimensions, we can take a simple 1 × 1 image (i.e., a file that takes virtually no time to download) and use it to create bars of any length or width of our choosing.

One of the nice features of CGI programming with Perl is Perl's ability integrate local variables and HTML code seamlessly into a program. We have

FIGURE 11.1. A gray bar generated by adjusting the WIDTH and HEIGHT attributes of a 1 × 1 gray pixel.

seen, for example, that we can use a command such as `print "Your name is $name"`, and Perl will substitute the actual content of the variable $name into the sentence. Conveniently, we can exploit this feature of Perl to create on-the-fly bar graphs. If we have two local variables that represent the means for two groups (e.g., $mean1 and $mean2), we can use those variables as attributes in the IMG tags to create bars of specific dimensions:

```
<IMG SRC='/images/bargray.jpg' WIDTH=$mean1
   HEIGHT='20'><BR>
<IMG SRC='/images/bargray.jpg' WIDTH=$mean2
   HEIGHT='20'><BR>
```

Let's study a working example. The script below, graphbar.pl, is designed to create a bar graph that summarizes the cell means from a 2 × 2 experiment. Before I explain how the program works, I want you to experiment a bit with the numbers so you can see how the program operates. Copy the two scripts below into blank documents and name them graphdemobar.pl and graphbar.pl respectively in your server's cgi-bin directory. (You'll likely have already downloaded all the images from my server and saved them to the images folder on your server; if you haven't you'll need to do so.) The script, graphdemobar.pl, is not an actual part of the graphing program. It simply provides an interface for the purposes of this demonstration.

graphdemobar.pl

```
#!C:/perl/bin/perl.exe
use CGI;
$query = new CGI;

print $query->header;
print $query->start_html(-title=>'Bar graph demo');
print "<FORM ACTION='/cgi-bin/graphbar.pl'
   METHOD='post'>";

print "Please enter the means for each cell of the
   design.<BR>";
print "Factor 1 Level 1, Factor 2 Level 1 <INPUT
   TYPE='textbox' NAME='m1' MAXLENGTH=3 SIZE=3><BR>";
print "Factor 1 Level 1, Factor 2 Level 2 <INPUT
   TYPE='textbox' NAME='m2' MAXLENGTH=3 SIZE=3><BR>";
print "Factor 1 Level 2, Factor 2 Level 1 <INPUT
   TYPE='textbox' NAME='m3' MAXLENGTH=3 SIZE=3><BR>";
```

```perl
print "Factor 1 Level 2, Factor 2 Level 2 <INPUT
   TYPE='textbox' NAME='m4' MAXLENGTH=3 SIZE=3><BR>";

print "<INPUT TYPE='submit'>";
print "</FORM>";
print $query->end_html;
```


graphbar.pl

```perl
#!C:/perl/bin/perl.exe
use CGI;
$query = new CGI;

$m1= $query->param('m1');
$m2= $query->param('m2');
$m3= $query->param('m3');
$m4= $query->param('m4');

$heightconstant=25;
#---------------------------
print $query->header;
print $query->start_html(-title=>'Bar graph demo');
print "<FONT FACE = 'arial' SIZE = '2'>";
print "<BR>";

# Create legend
print "<TABLE><TR>";
print "<TR><TD><FONT FACE = 'arial' SIZE = '2'>
   <B>Factor 2</B></TD></TR>";
print "<TD><FONT FACE = 'arial' SIZE = '2'><IMG
   SRC='/images/bargray.jpg' WIDTH='10' HEIGHT= '10'>
   Level 1 </TD></TR>";
print "<TD><FONT FACE = 'arial' SIZE = '2'><IMG
   SRC='/images/barblack.jpg' WIDTH='10' HEIGHT= '10'>
   Level 2 </TD></TR>";
print "</TABLE>";

# Create bars
print "<TABLE><TR>";
$tall= $m1*$heightconstant;
print "<TD VALIGN='bottom' ALIGN='center'
   BGCOLOR='#F8F8F8'>
<FONT FACE = 'arial' SIZE = '2'>$m1 <BR>
<IMG SRC='/images/bargray.jpg' WIDTH='40' HEIGHT=
   $tall></TD>";
```

```
$tall= $m2*$heightconstant;
print "<TD VALIGN='bottom' ALIGN='center'
   BGCOLOR='#F8F8F8'>
<FONT FACE = 'arial' SIZE = '2'>$m2 <BR>
<IMG SRC='/images/barblack.jpg' WIDTH='40' HEIGHT=
   $tall></TD>";

$tall= $m3*$heightconstant;
print "<TD VALIGN='bottom' ALIGN='center'
   BGCOLOR='#F8F8F8'>
<FONT FACE = 'arial' SIZE = '2'>$m3 <BR>
<IMG SRC='/images/bargray.jpg' WIDTH='40' HEIGHT=
   $tall></TD>";

$tall= $m4*$heightconstant;
print "<TD VALIGN='bottom' ALIGN='center'
   BGCOLOR='#F8F8F8'>
<FONT FACE = 'arial' SIZE = '2'>$m4 <BR>
<IMG SRC='/images/barblack.jpg' WIDTH='40'
   HEIGHT=$tall></TD>";
print "</TR>";

print "<TR>
<TD COLSPAN=2 BGCOLOR='#F8F8F8' ALIGN='center'><FONT
   FACE = 'arial' SIZE = '2'> Level 1 </TD>
<TD COLSPAN=2 BGCOLOR='#F8F8F8' ALIGN='center'><FONT
   FACE = 'arial' SIZE = '2'> Level 2 </TD>
</TR>";
print "<TR>
<TD COLSPAN=4 BGCOLOR='330066' ALIGN='center'><FONT
   FACE = 'arial' SIZE = '2' COLOR='white'> <B>Factor
   1</B> </TD>
</TR>";
print "</TABLE>";

print $query->end_html;
```

When you enter the URL for the interface script, graphdemobar.pl, into your browser window you should see a page like the one illustrated in Figure 11.2.

Type in some means for the four conditions of a hypothetical 2 × 2 experiment. When you press **Submit**, you should see a bar graph, such as the one shown in Figure 11.3, that visually depicts those means. Play around with a variety of different values so you can see how the program operates.

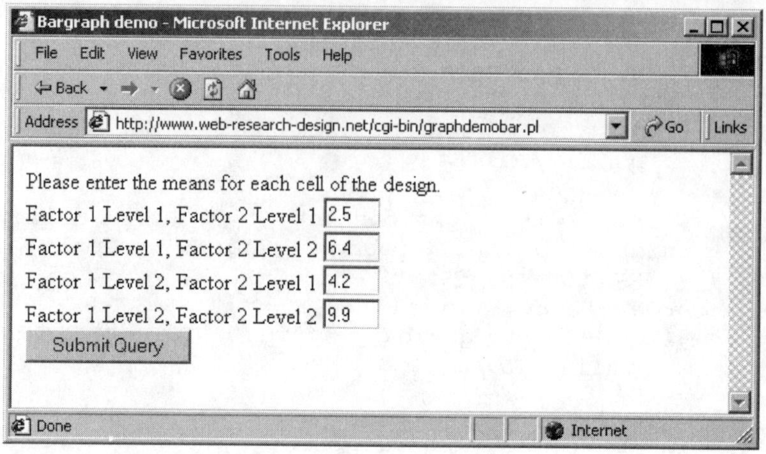

FIGURE 11.2. The interface page for the bar graph script.

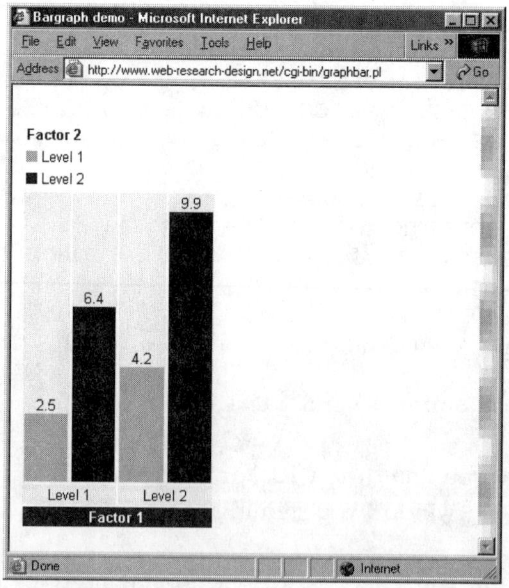

FIGURE 11.3. An example of a bar graph generated by tweaking the dimensions of simple images in Perl.

The first file creates a simple interface web page designed to facilitate the demonstration by obtaining some values for graphing; the second script, **graphbar.pl**, is the one that actually creates the graphs. In your research, you'll probably have a script that opens a data file and calculates the cell means. You then would want to pass those means, via hidden tags, to graphbar.pl (or a modified version of graphbar.pl) to have them graphed.

Let's study the code for graphbar.pl. The first major thing the program does is read the values for the cell means from the submitted data packet. Those cell means are assigned the names $m1, $m2, $m3, and $m4. Next, the program creates a table and simply places an image in each cell of the table, making the image's height as large as the value of the corresponding cell mean. The rest of the code is just simple formatting designed to make the graph look nice. For example, we have used the ALIGN attribute to align the bars along the bottom of their cells.

One thing we have done that might seem a bit unusual at first is that we have taken the cell means and multiplied them by a constant named $heightconstant: `$tall= $m1*$heightconstant`. In this example, $heightconstant was set to 25. Because the cell means will represent the height of the bars in the metric of pixels, it will be difficult to see the bars if they are only 3 pixels high, for example. (Recall that the original image, which is only 1 pixel high, was almost impossible to see.) If we multiply the means by a constant, we can make the bars taller without distorting the relationships among the means.

Notice that we've only used two images in this graph: bargray.jpg and barblack.jpg. The fact that only two very small image files are involved helps the page load quickly.

If you want to use this script to summarize the results of your studies for your participants, here are a few things you'll need to do:

- Before calling the script (i.e., activating the script), you'll need to have computed the cell means in your sample. We discussed methods for reading data from a file and averaging scores in Chapter 6.
- If the cell means submitted to graphbar.pl do not have names such as m1, m2, m3, and m4, you'll need to alter the $query->param tags at the top of graphbar.pl so that they are bringing in the correct values.
- You'll need to customize the text within and around the graph. I've used the labels "Factor 1," "Level 1," and so on in this example. Obviously you

would replace them with labels that are more descriptive. Also, it would be helpful to include some text that helps explain what the results mean. You can create verbal summaries of the many possible patterns of data that could be observed and, via if–then conditionals, print the appropriate one.

- If you want to expand the program to represent the means for, say, a 2×3 experiment, you can do so easily by adding new lines to the code.

In summary, we can create bar graphs on-the-fly by substituting local variables for the heights or widths of simple image files. The script presented here is sufficiently generic that you should be able to adopt it easily to suit your needs.

TWO-DIMENSIONAL COORDINATE GRAPHS

Another kind of graph that can be useful for summarizing a participant's data—especially in individual differences research—is a two-dimensional coordinate graph. Let's assume, for example, that you had measured two variables, Extraversion and Neuroticism, and you wanted to show your user where he or she was located in the two-dimensional space defined by these variables.

The generic script below, graph2d.pl, can be used to plot a person's score in two-dimensional space. Copy it to a blank document and save it as graph2d.pl to your server's cgi-bin directory. For the purpose of illustrating how the program works, you'll also need to copy the demonstration interface: graphdemo2d.pl and save it to your server's cgi-bin directory.

graphdemo2d.pl

```
#!C:/perl/bin/perl.exe
use CGI;
$query = new CGI;

print $query->header;
print $query->start_html(-title=>'2D Graph Demo');
print "<FORM ACTION='/cgi-bin/graph2d.pl'
   METHOD='post'>";
print "<FONT FACE = 'arial' SIZE = '2'>";
print "Two-dimensional graphing demo.<BR>";
```

```
print "Please enter the x and y coordinates for the
   point you'd like to plot.<BR>";
print "x <INPUT TYPE='textbox' NAME='xcoord'
   MAXLENGTH=3 SIZE=3><BR>";
print "y <INPUT TYPE='textbox' NAME='ycoord'
   MAXLENGTH=3 SIZE=3><BR><BR>";

print "Please enter the minimum and maximum possible
   values of these variables.<BR>";
print "min <INPUT TYPE='textbox' NAME='xmin'
   MAXLENGTH=3 SIZE=3><BR>";
print "max <INPUT TYPE='textbox' NAME='xmax'
   MAXLENGTH=3 SIZE=3><BR>";

print "<INPUT TYPE='submit'>";
print "</FORM>";
print $query->end_html;
```

---

graph2d.pl

```perl
#!C:/perl/bin/perl.exe
use CGI;
$query = new CGI;

$xcoord= $query->param('xcoord');
$ycoord= $query->param('ycoord');
$xmin= $query->param('xmin');
$xmax= $query->param('xmax');

#--------------------------

$b = (17/($xmax - $xmin));
$a = -1*($b*$xmin);

$xcoordnew= $a + $b*$xcoord;
$ycoordnew= $a + $b*$ycoord;

$xcoordnew = sprintf("%.0f", $xcoordnew);
$ycoordnew = sprintf("%.0f", $ycoordnew);

#--------------------------

print $query->header;
print $query->start_html(-title=>'2D Graph Demo');
print "<FONT FACE = 'arial' SIZE = '2'>";
```

```
print "<CENTER>";
print "<TABLE background='/images/2dback360.jpg'
   border='0' cellspacing='0' cellpadding='0'>";

for($y = 0; $y <= 17;++$y){
   print "<TR>";
      for($x = 0; $x <= 17; ++$x){
      print "<TD>";
      if($xcoordnew == $x && $ycoordnew ==$y){
        print "<IMG SRC='/images/dot.gif'>";
      }
    else{
        print "<IMG SRC='/images/blank.gif'>";
      }
    print "</TD>";
      }
print "</TR>";
}
print "</TABLE>";
print "</CENTER>";

print "Original (x, y) coordinates: ($xcoord,
   $ycoord)<BR>";
print "Transformed coordinates: ($xcoordnew,
   $ycoordnew)<BR>";

print $query->end_html;
```

To see what the program does, run the demonstration file, graphdemo2d.pl. You should see something like the screen illustrated in Figure 11.4.

Enter an *x* (vertical) and a *y* (horizontal) coordinate for the point you wish to plot. Also, enter the minimum and maximum values for the dimensions. If, for example, your variables were measured on a 1 to 7 metric, you would enter 1 for "min" and 7 for "max." This program assumes that both scales are measured in the same metric; if this is not a reasonable assumption, the program can be easily modified to accommodate differences in scale.

When you submit your query, you should see a graph similar to the one shown in Figure 11.5. Notice that a two-dimensional space is depicted, and an × has been placed in the appropriate location of the space. We have used the midpoint of both scales, a value of 4, as the origin for this graph. Therefore,

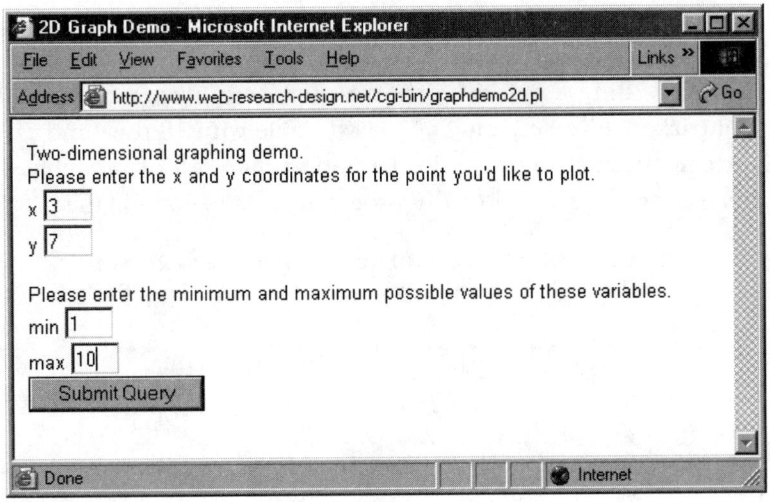

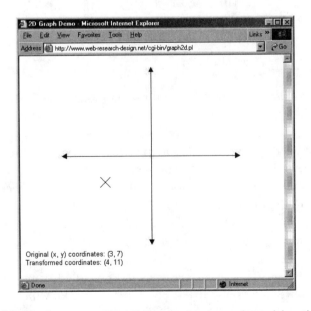

FIGURE 11.4. The interface page for the two-dimensional coordinate plot script.

FIGURE 11.5. An example of the output produced by the two-dimensional coordinate plotting script.

the two axes intersect at the coordinate (4, 4) rather than (0, 0) (the common origin in algebraic texts).

How did we pull this off? We employed three tricks here. The first critical trick involved creating an HTML table with 18 rows and 18 columns, and placing an image of an × in the appropriate cell of the table. Let's begin by dissecting the section of the program responsible for this:

```
print "<TABLE background='/images/2dback360.jpg'
   border='0' cellspacing='0' cellpadding='0'>";

for($y = 0; $y <= 17;++$y){
    print "<TR>";
        for($x = 0; $x <= 17; ++$x){
            print "<TD>";
            if($xcoordnew == $x && $ycoordnew ==$y){
                print "<IMG SRC='/images/dot.gif'>";
            }
            else{
                print "<IMG SRC='/images/blank.gif'>";
            }
        print "</TD>";
    }
print "</TR>";
}
print "</TABLE>";
```

Notice that we've created two for-next loops. The first, which uses the index value $y, is used to create the rows. The second, which uses the index value $x, is used to create each cell within a row. By nesting one loop within the other, we've created a situation in which we create a row, create 18 cells within that row, then move on to the next row until we've created 18 rows.

What is particularly noteworthy here is that, as each cell of the table is created, the program decides, via if–else conditions, whether the coordinates of the current cell (indexed by $x and $y) are equal to the coordinates of the point to be plotted. If so, then the program inserts an image of an × called dot.gif into that cell of the table. If not, then the program inserts a blank image of the same dimensions as dot.gif called blank.gif.

We've just seen the second major trick, which involves the use of precreated images. There are three image files associated with this graph: dot.gif, blank.gif, and 2dback360.jpg. dot.gif is a 20 × 20 pixel image of a cross (i.e., ×). blank.gif is a 20 × 20 pixel image of nothing. 2dback360.jpg is a 360 × 360 pixel image that depicts the two axes. In the TABLE tag, we've instructed the browser to use this image as the background for the table. (This command only works in Microsoft's Internet Explorer; the background image does not appear in Netscape. In the next section I'll show you how to design a 2-D coordinate plot that doesn't require any images so that you don't alienate your subjects who are using Netscape.)

To ensure that the table and the image will have identical dimensions, we've programmed the for–next loops to create 18 cells (0 to 17) in each of the 18 rows. We'll be placing a 20 × 20 pixel image within each cell. By doing this 18 times in each direction, we'll be ensuring that the table itself is (18 × 20) = 360 pixels in width and height, thereby matching the dimensions of the background image.

Both dot.gif and blank.gif were created with a "transparent" background. As a result, when these images are placed on top of the background image (2dback360.jpg in this case), you can still see the background image through the empty space of the new image. Thus, when we place blank.gif in each unoccupied cell of the table, we're not actually covering up the background image. blank.gif is kind of like a 20 × 20 piece of glass, and we use it simply to ensure that the cell will be the right size.

The third trick involves mapping the metric of the variables to a metric appropriate for the table. Recall that the table is set up to create 18 × 18 cells. Thus, the *x* and *y* coordinates for the table range between 0 and 17. We need to take the metric of our variables and transform them to a 0 to 17 metric and, in the process, remap the data point we wish to plot to this new metric.

The following code does just that:

```
$b  =  (17/($xmax  -  $xmin));
$a  =  -1*($b*$xmin);

$xcoordnew= $a  +  $b*$xcoord;
$ycoordnew= $a  +  $b*$ycoord;

$xcoordnew  =  sprintf("%.0f,"  $xcoordnew);
$ycoordnew  =  sprintf("%.0f,"  $ycoordnew);
```

To see how this code works, assume that we were working with variables that were measured in a metric that ranges from 1 to 10. We need to map the minimum possible value of 1 on the original metric to the minimum possible value of 0 in the table metric. Similarly, we need to map the maximum possible value of 10 in the original metric to the maximum possible value of 17 in the table metric. This is a simple problem in linear algebra that should be familiar to any researcher who uses linear regression. We're trying to find a line of form $y = a + b \times x$ that connects these two points, as illustrated in Figure 11.6. To do so, we construct the following linear equations:

$$0 = a + b \times 1$$

$$17 = a + b \times 10$$

and solve them for a and b. To do so, let's first express both of them with respect to a:

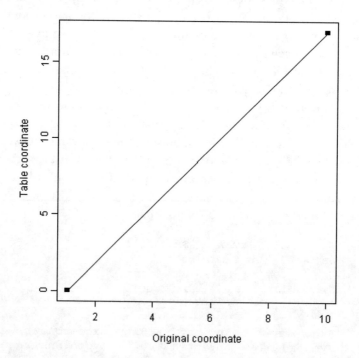

FIGURE 11.6. We are trying to find an equation that will allow us to map each original coordinate onto the dimensions of the table.

$$a = -b \times 1$$

$$a = 17 - b \times 10$$

If we set these two terms equal to one another, we obtain $(-b \times 1) = (17 - b \times 10)$. We can now solve for b. $b(-1 + 10) = 17$ or $b = (17/9)$. We can now take this value of b and substitute it into one of our original equations and solve for a. If we do this with the first equation, we obtain $0 = a + (17/9) \times 1$ or $a = -17/9$. Thus, the linear equation that maps the values from our original 1 to 10 metric to the table 0 to 17 metric is:

Table coordinate $= -(17/9) + (17/9) \times$ Original coordinate.

We can take any coordinate in its original 1 to 10 metric and use this equation to determine the coordinates for the table cell in which it should be plotted. I've been using the coordinates 3, 7. Notice that if we use the equation above to map the x coordinate, 3, onto the table's x metric, we obtain a value of 3.77, which we round up to 4. Using the same equation, we see that the value of 7 in the original y metric maps to 11.33, which rounds down to 11 in the table's y metric. The final coordinates for the point in the table's metric are (4, 11). The point will be plotted in the cell of the table in which $x equals 4 and $y equals 11.

Notice that the form of the solution is general, and the programming code takes advantage of that. In other words, you don't need to work out the mathematics each time you want to use a new metric. By providing the program with the minimum and maximum values of the original variables, the program automatically determines the appropriate mapping between the original metric and the table metric.

To adopt this program for your use, you'll need to do the following:

- After calculating a person's score on two dimensions, you'll need to pass these two values via hidden tags to the graph2d.pl script.
- You'll need either to (1) tell the script, via hidden tags, the minimum and maximum values of the scales or (2) assign these values to variables in graph2d.pl without reading the values in as CGI data.
- Notice that the graph2d.pl script reads the values from $query assuming they are named *xcoord* and *ycoord*, respectively. If these are not the names you used in your program, you'll need to enter the appropriate names here. For

example, if you used *neuroticsmscore* and *extraversionscore*, you'll need to modify these statements to read: $xcoord= $query->param('neuroticism score') and $ycoord= $query-> param('extraversion score').

It is also possible to create a two-dimensional coordinate graph with no prefabricated graphics files whatsoever. For example, try replacing the for-next codes in the graph2d.pl script with the following:

graph2dsimple.pl

```
print "<CENTER>";
print "<TABLE border='1' BORDERCOLOR='lightblue'
   cellspacing='0' cellpadding='0'>";
for($y = 17; $y >= 0; --$y){
   print "<TR>";
   for($x = 0; $x <= 17; ++$x){
      print "<TD WIDTH='20' HEIGHT='10' ALIGN='center'>";
      if($xcoordnew == $x && $ycoordnew ==$y){
      print "<B>X</B>";
   }
      else{
         if($y == 0){
            $labelx = $xmin + (($xmax-$xmin)/17)*$x;
            $labelx = sprintf("%.1f," $labelx);
            print "$labelx";
         }
         if($x == 0 && $y != 0){
            $labely = $xmin + (($xmax-$xmin)/17)*$y;
            $labely = sprintf("%.1f," $labely);
            print "$labely";
         }
         if($x != 0 && $y != 0){
            print "   ";
         }
      }
   print "</TD>";
   }
print "</TR>";
}
print "</TABLE>";
print "</CENTER>";
```

Save the new file as graph2dsimple.pl in your server's cgi-bin directory. Also, modify graphdemo2d.pl so that it activates graph2dsimple.pl and save the graphdemo2dsimple.pl modified file as graphdemo2dsimple.pl in your server's cgi-bin folder. Run graphdemo2dsimple.pl in your browser.

The resulting graph uses the same table techniques, but does not use a background image. Moreover, instead of inserting an image to represent the data point, the program inserts a simple piece of text: an X. Finally, it uses the BORDERS attribute of the table, as well as the BORDERCOLOR attribute, to create a graphing paper-like appearance. Figure 11.7 illustrates such a graph using the coordinates (3, 7), with minimum and maximum values of 1 and 10 respectively. This method for producing two-dimensional coordinate plots is more safe if you want to ensure that the graph will appear correctly on a variety of browsers.

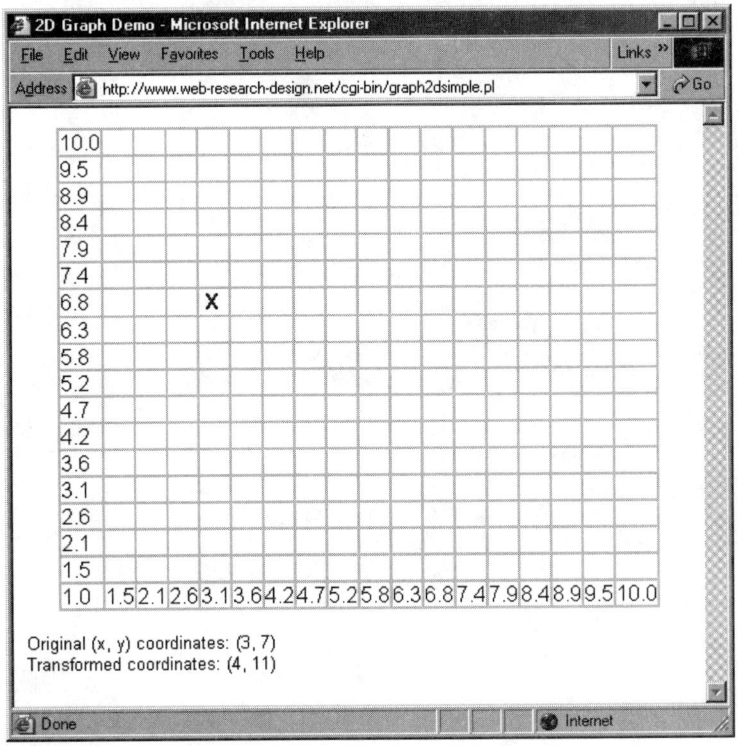

FIGURE 11.7. An example of a coordinate plot that does not require the use of images.

> **Note.** In the for–next loop indexed by $y, notice that instead of counting from 0 to 17, we're counting backwards from 17 to 0. We accomplish this by (1) using --$y instead of ++$y in the for–next command and (2) starting with a counting value that is higher than the ending value. This allows us to order the values on the vertical axis from highest to lowest.

SUMMARY

In this chapter you have learned techniques for creating graphs that summarize the data for yourself and your participants. These generic scripts can be modified easily to accommodate different kinds of research projects.

Chapter 12

Tracking Participants over Multiple Sessions

PINs, Passwords, and Menus

One reason the Internet is a useful tool for behavioral research is that it provides an effective way to study people over repeated sessions. If you were interested in measuring people's political attitudes over time, for example, you could ask subjects to visit your site to complete attitude measures once a week for several consecutive weeks. By participating online, your participants could log-on at their convenience, and the data can be automatically time-stamped and stored by the server.

In order to keep the same person's data from different measurement sessions organized, you can assign your participants **Personal Identification Numbers** (PINs). PINs can be used to keep one person's data distinct from those of another. Moreover, you can use PINs to match a participant's data when merging data files from different sessions. In short, PINs are a useful tool for keeping people's data from multiple sessions linked.

AN EXAMPLE

To illustrate the way that PINs can be used to organize a subject's responses to multiple sessions, please visit the following web page on my server: http://www.web-research-design.net/cgi-bin/pindemo1.pl. The first page you'll see will ask you for your PIN and password (see Figure 12.1). For the purposes of this demonstration, enter a number between 100 and 200 for your PIN and use *web* as your password. (You can try it on your server after seeing how it works on my own.) This particular demonstration takes advantage of PINs in order to break a larger survey into smaller components. By doing so, you can make sure the data are saved on a section-by-section basis. This will help avoid problems that might occur when users need to end their participation prematurely due to fatigue or dial-up disconnects.

After you've entered your PIN and password, you'll be taken to a new page. This page has a menu that lists four component surveys (i.e., "Background Information," "Political Attitudes," "Personality," "Relationships"; see Figure 12.2) that are part of a larger study. The menu also indicates which of these surveys you've taken thus far. At this point you haven't taken any of the surveys, so each survey should be listed as "Not completed" in the status column. Now take the first survey by clicking the **Next Survey** button.

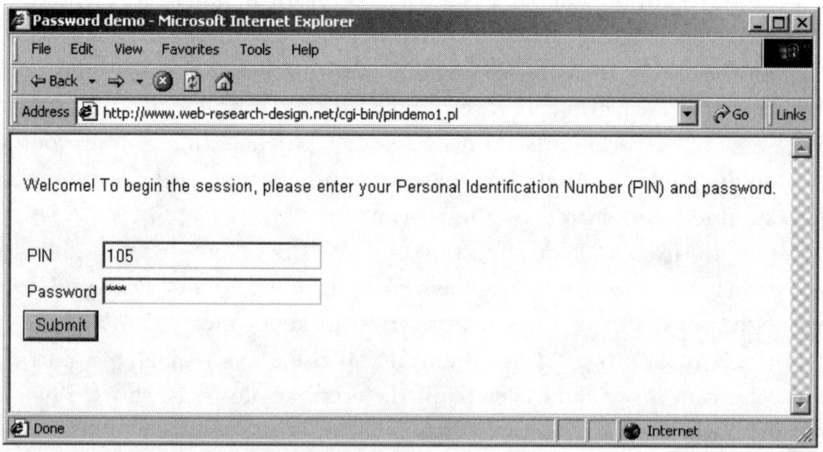

FIGURE 12.1. The login page.

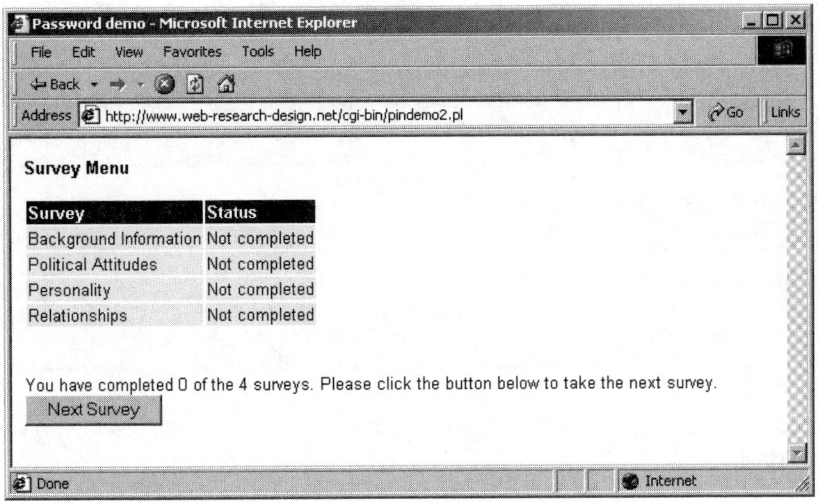

FIGURE 12.2. This menu welcomes the participant and shows which surveys or experiments have or have not been completed.

To conserve space, I have deliberately not included real surveys in this demonstration. Thus, when you go to a survey page, you'll see a screen like the one illustrated in Figure 12.3. Pretend that you just completed a questionnaire, and click the **Submit Data** button. You will now be taken back to the main menu. Notice that the menu now has you listed as having taken the first survey. If you continue to take more surveys, this menu will continue to update itself, as illustrated in Figure 12.4. Therefore, if you need to leave at any point, you can do so and return by going to the login page (i.e., http://www.web-research-design.net/cgi-bin/pindemo1.pl) and picking up where you left off. Once you've taken all four surveys, the menu screen will tell you that you have finished.

DISSECTING THE CODE

Now that you have a sense of how the program works, let's see how the CGI scripts accomplish this. There are several scripts involved in this program. Here is a brief overview.

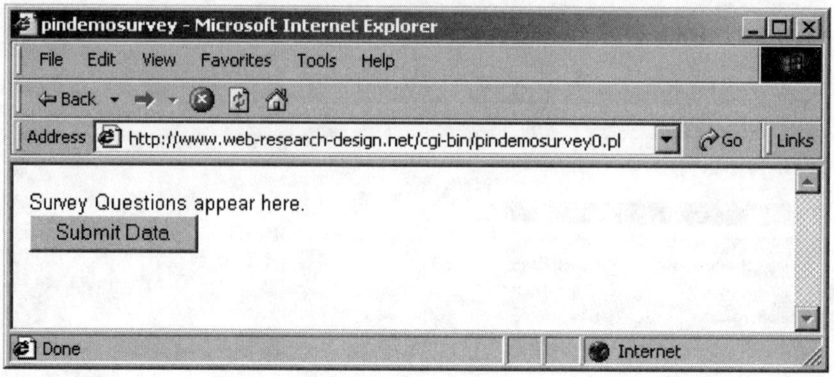

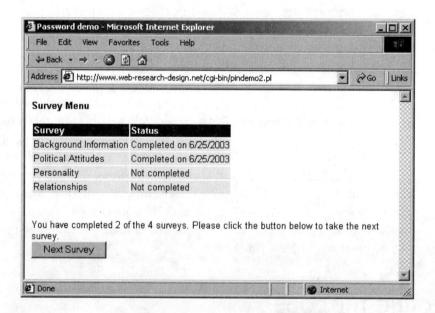

FIGURE 12.3. In an actual study, the survey questions would appear on this page.

FIGURE 12.4. After the user has completed a survey, the menu page updates itself and shows the user which surveys have been completed and when they were completed.

- pindemo1.pl This script is responsible for obtaining the PIN and password from the user. The PIN and password are passed on to pindemo2.pl via hidden tags.
- pindemo2.pl This script is responsible for a number of tasks. First, it checks the PIN and password against a pre-existing text file data base (passwords.txt) to see if they are legitimate. If so, pindemo2.pl creates a menu of the various surveys. In creating this menu, the script opens and reads a text file called participation.txt to determine which surveys the user has completed. It uses this information to update the "Status" section of the menu. When the user clicks on the **Next Survey** button, one of the following four scripts is activated:
- pindemosurvey0.pl–pindemosurvey3.pl These four scripts contain the four questionnaires. For the purposes of this demonstration, there aren't any real survey questions in these four files. These dummy scripts read in the user's PIN and password, and pass them on to the next script that is activated.
- pindemosave.pl This script is activated once the responses to a survey have been submitted. This script uses a generic set of commands to save the data into a file that is appropriate for the given survey. It also adds the user's PIN to the file so the various data sets can be merged easily once the project is complete. Finally, the script updates a text file called participation.txt that keeps track of which surveys the subject has completed.

Here is the actual code for the various scripts. Copy-and-paste these scripts to the cgi-bin of your server. Before these scripts will work properly on your server, you will also need to create a text file that contains password information. I'll explain how to do this after I walk you through some of the code.

pindemo1.pl

```
#!C:/perl/bin/perl.exe
use CGI;
$query = new CGI;

print $query->header;
print $query->start_html(-title=>'Password demo');

print "<FONT FACE = 'arial' SIZE = '2'>";
print "<FORM ACTION = '/cgi-bin/pindemo2.pl' METHOD =
    'post'> ";
print "<BR>Welcome! To begin the session, please enter
```

```
    your Personal Identification Number (PIN) and
    password. </B><BR><BR>";
print "<TABLE>
<TR>
<TD><FONT FACE = 'arial' SIZE = '2'> PIN</TD>
<TD> <INPUT TYPE='textbox' NAME='pin' SIZE='25'
    MAXLENGTH='30'></TD>
</TR>
<TR>
<TD><FONT FACE = 'arial' SIZE = '2'> Password </TD>
<TD> <INPUT TYPE='password' NAME='password' SIZE='25'
    MAXLENGTH='30'></TD>
</TR>
</TABLE>";

print "<INPUT TYPE='submit' VALUE='Submit'>";
print "</FORM>";
print $query->end_html;
```

This first script asks the user for his or her PIN and password using a *password text box*, which displays asterisks when the user types to prevent over-the-shoulder observation of the password.

Note. This is the first time we've discussed the **password text box** in this book. The general HTML code for this special type of text box is:

```
<INPUT TYPE='password' NAME='name' MAXLENGTH='30'
SIZE='25'>
```

This tag functions in the same way as a textbox tag, with two exceptions. First, the text typed into the box is replaced in its display on the screen by asterisks or dots so that casual observers cannot see the password as the user enters it. Second, the password is eliminated from the textbox as soon as the user submits the information, which means that another user cannot simply use the **back** button on the browser to return to the password page and discover the password.

The PIN and password are passed on to the next script, **pindemo2.pl**, via hidden tags when the **Submit** button is pressed. Here is the code for pindemo2.pl.

pindemo2.pl

```
#!C:/perl/bin/perl.exe
use CGI;
```

```perl
$query = new CGI;

print $query->header;
print $query->start_html(-title=>'Password demo');
print "<FONT FACE = 'arial' SIZE = '2'>";
#----------------------------------------------
$pin= $query->param('pin');
$password= $query->param('password');
$match= 0;

$v0 = "Background Information";
$v1 = "Political Attitudes";
$v2 = "Personality";
$v3 = "Relationships";
$numsurveys= 4;

#----------------------------------------------
open(INFO,
   "$ENV{'DOCUMENT_ROOT'}/www/data/passwords.txt");
@passdata = <INFO>;
close(INFO);
#----------------------------------------------

foreach $key (@passdata)
{
   ($pin2,$storedpassword,$e)=split(/,/,$key);
   if( ($pin eq $pin2) && ($password eq
     $storedpassword) )
   {
     $match= 1;
   }
}
#----------------------------------------------

if ($match == 0)
{
   print "Invalid response. <BR><BR>";
   print "If you think you may have made a typo,
     please click your browser's <I>Back</I> button
     and try again. <BR><BR>";
}
#----------------------------------------------

if ($match == 1)
{
```

```perl
    print "<B>Survey Menu</B><BR><BR>";
    open(INFO,
        "$ENV{'DOCUMENT_ROOT'}/www/data/participation.txt");
    @participation = <INFO>;
    close(INFO);

$tasks = 0;
@dates = ();
foreach $key (@participation)
{
    ($pin2,$section,$date)=split(/,/,$key);
    if($pin2 eq $pin)
    {
    $tasks= $tasks + 1;
    @dates = (@dates, $date);
    }
}

print "<TABLE>";
print "<TR BGCOLOR='darkblue'>
<TD><FONT FACE='arial' SIZE='2'
    COLOR='white'><B>Survey</B></TD>
<TD><FONT FACE='arial' SIZE='2'
    COLOR='white'><B>Status</B></TD>
</TR>";

for($i = 0; $i <= ($numsurveys - 1); ++$i)
{
$listing = "v" . $i;
    print "<TR BGCOLOR='beige'>
    <TD><FONT FACE='arial' SIZE='2'>$$listing</TD>";

    if($i < $tasks){
        print "<TD><FONT FACE='arial' SIZE='2'>Completed
            on $dates[$i]</TD>";
    }
    else{
    print "<TD><FONT FACE='arial' SIZE='2'>Not
        completed</TD>";
    }
print "</TR>";
}
print "</TABLE>";

    if($tasks < $numsurveys){
```

```
    $nextaction = "/cgi-bin/" . "pindemosurvey" .
        $tasks . ".pl";
    print "<FORM ACTION=$nextaction METHOD='post'>";
    print "<INPUT TYPE='hidden' NAME='pin'
        VALUE=$pin>";
    print "<INPUT TYPE='hidden' NAME='password'
        VALUE=$password>";
    print "<BR>You have completed $tasks of the 4
        surveys. Please click the button below to take
        the next survey.<BR>";
    print "<INPUT TYPE='submit' VALUE='Next
        Survey'>";
    print "</FORM>";
    }
 if($tasks >= $numsurveys){
 print "<BR>You have completed all the
     questionnaires.<BR><BR>Debriefing.";
  }
}

print $query->end_html;
```

The first thing this script does is read in the values for the PIN and password from the submitted CGI data packet. These values are assigned to the local variables $pin and $password, respectively.

The next task is to determine whether the PIN and password are legitimate. To do so, the script opens the text file **passwords.txt** in the **data** folder of the server and assigns the contents to the array @passdata. The contexts of **password.txt** look something like this:

```
100,web,endline
101,web,endline
102,web,endline
103,web,endline
104,web,endline
```

The first element in each row contains a legitimate PIN. The second value contains the password corresponding to that particular PIN. (In this example, all the passwords are identical.) The third value is simply a placeholder that denotes the last element of the row. In order for the CGI scripts to function appropriately on your server, you'll need to create a new file in your text editor, enter some data similar to those above, and save the file as a text file in the data folder of your server. You can use the same usernames and passwords as I have used here, or you can create your own list of usernames and passwords. (You can also make the passwords unique to each username.)

In the next segment of the script, the program loops through each line of @passdata, assigns the three values to temporary variables (i.e., $pin2, $storedpassword, and $e). If the value of $pin2 equals $pin *and* if the value of $password equals $storedpassword, the program assigns the value of 1 to $match. Thus, if the user has entered a valid PIN and a valid password corresponding to that PIN, the value of $match is set to 1. If not, the value of $match equals 0.

In the next segment of code, the program determines whether or not $match equals 0. If $match equals 0, the program prints an error message for the user. If $match equals 1, the program moves onto the next big task: creating a menu of survey options.

Recall that the menu is customized; it indicates which of the surveys the user has completed and when those surveys were completed. To determine this information, the script opens a text file called participation.txt. This file may look something like this:

```
100,0,4/15/2002
100,1,4/15/2002
100,2,4/15/2002
101,0,4/20/2002
102,0,4/21/2002
101,1,4/22/2002
102,1,4/23/2002
```

In short, each line contains a record of *any* participation on the part of a user. (You do not need to create the participation.txt file on your server; the pindemosave.pl script will create the file automatically the first time it is needed.) There are three pieces of information per line. The first is the PIN of the person who completed a survey. The second is the survey number that the participant completed. The third is the date for which the survey was submitted. Using a loop, the script reads each line of these data and assigns the values to temporary variables: $pin2, $section, and $date. While cycling through this loop, the program checks to see whether the value of $pin2 is equal to the current person's PIN (i.e., $pin). If so, the program increments the value of $tasks by 1.

Notice that $tasks starts at 0 and gets incremented by one each time the program finds a record for participation. The program will use this information to determine which survey the person needs to complete next. What happens as a result of this process? If the person's PIN were 100 in this example, the value of tasks when the loop is complete will be 3. (The program begins with a $tasks value of 0 and increments that by 1 each time it finds a record [three times] for subject 100 in the participation.txt file.) If the person's PIN were 102, the value of tasks when the loop is complete will be 2.

The next significant portion of code creates the table and lists the various surveys within. Using if-else conditions, the code determines whether to tag a survey as Completed or Not completed. If the survey has been completed, the code lists the date at on which the survey data were submitted. This has been read into an array called @dates in the previous loop. Finally, the user is provided with a **Submit** button that enables him or her to take the next survey.

The program uses the value of $tasks to determine which of the four surveys is to be administered next. If $tasks equals 2, the program will activate pindemosurvey2.pl when the **Submit** button is clicked. Notice that we've used some Perl tricks for appending strings (see Chapter 9) in order to create the necessary URL:

```
$nextaction = "/cgi-bin/" . "pindemosurvey" . $tasks . ".pl";
```

We've essentially inserted the value of $tasks into the URL in just the right place. By substituting $nextaction for our ACTION attribute in the FORM tag, we can ensure that the user will be taken to the next appropriate survey when he or she clicks the **Submit** button.

Notice that these commands are only executed if $tasks is less than 4. If $tasks equals 4, then the user has completed all the surveys. An if–else condition is used to determine whether this is the case, and a concluding message is presented if all the tasks are complete.

The next script is pindemosurvey0.pl—the first of the four surveys. As I mentioned before, I did not actually insert survey items into this script. I've left that part to you. I have, however, included some features that are necessary for making the larger program work effectively. Here is the code:

pindemosurvey0.pl

```
#!C:/perl/bin/perl.exe
use CGI;
$query = new CGI;

$pin= $query->param('pin');
$password= $query->param('password');

print $query->header;
print $query->start_html(-title=>'pindemosurvey');
print "<FORM ACTION = '/cgi-bin/pindemosave.pl' METHOD
   = 'post'> ";


print "<FONT FACE = 'arial' SIZE = '2'>";

print "Survey Questions appear here. <BR>";

print "<INPUT TYPE='hidden' NAME='survey' VALUE='0'>";
print "<INPUT TYPE='hidden' NAME='pin' VALUE=$pin>";
print "<INPUT TYPE='hidden' NAME='password'
   VALUE=$password>";
print "<INPUT TYPE = 'submit' VALUE = 'Submit
   Data'>";
print "</FORM></FONT>";
print $query->end_html;
```

The script reads in the values of $pin and $password. Importantly, it passes those values along when the **Submit** button is pressed. Recall that the interaction between the user and the server is stateless (see Chapter 9). If we don't carry the user's PIN and password forward in this manner, the server will forget the fact that it is interacting with the same user with whom it was previously interacting. Notice that we've also created a hidden value called "survey" that corresponds to which survey is being presented. This is used by the next script, which is responsible for saving the data.

pindemosave.pl is activated whenever a user submits data from one of the four surveys. Here is the code:

pindemosave.pl

```
#!C:/perl/bin/perl.exe
use CGI;
$query = new CGI;
```

```
$pin= $query->param('pin');
$password= $query->param('password');
$survey= $query->param('survey');

$filename = ">>$ENV{'DOCUMENT_ROOT'}/www/data/" .
   "pindata" . $survey . ".txt";
($sec,$min,$hour,$mday,$mon,$year,$wday,$yday,$isdst) =
   localtime(time);
$year=$year+1900;

open(INFO, $filename);
   print INFO "$pin, ";
   print INFO "$mon/$mday/$year, ";
   print INFO "$hour:$min:$sec, ";
   foreach $key (sort($query->param))
      {
      $value = $query->param($key);
      print INFO "$value, ";
      }
   print INFO "endline \n";
close(INFO);

open(INFO,
   ">>$ENV{'DOCUMENT_ROOT'}/www/data/participation.txt")
   ;
print INFO "$pin, $survey, $mon/$mday/$year \n";
close(INFO);

print $query->header;
print $query->start_html(-title=>'Password demo');

print "<FONT FACE = 'arial' SIZE = '2'>";
print "<FORM ACTION = '/cgi-bin/pindemo2.pl' METHOD =
   'post'> ";
print "<INPUT TYPE='hidden' NAME='pin' VALUE=$pin>";
print "<INPUT TYPE='hidden' NAME='password'
   VALUE=$password>";
print "Thank you. Your data have been saved.<BR><BR>";
print "<INPUT TYPE='submit' VALUE='Return to menu'>";
print "</FORM>";
print $query->end_html;
```

This program contains a chunk of code designed to save the data from the survey in a generic way:

```
foreach $key (sort($query->param))
    {
    $value = $query->param($key);
    print INFO "$value, ";
    }
```

In other words, the program is naïve to the actual variables in question; it simply saves whatever information it receives to the appropriate data file. As a general rule, you shouldn't use this method to save your data because it will not show you when nonresponses have occurred. Instead, you should save your data by explicitly reading each variable from the CGI data packet and printing it to the data file, as we've done in previous examples. I've included this approach here simply because we haven't included actual stimuli and, as a consequence, haven't defined explicit variables.

How does the script know which survey file to save the data from? Recall that we passed a hidden value called "survey" to this script from the survey itself. The value of that variable is used to determine where to save the data. Taking advantage of Perl's ability to append variables and text, we insert the value of $survey into the filename to which we want the data saved:

```
$filename = ">>$ENV{'DOCUMENT_ROOT'}/www/data/" .
    "pindata" . $survey . ".txt";
```

Thus, if the value of $survey is 0, we are assigning $ENV{'DOCUMENT_ROOT'}/www/data/pindata0.txt to the variable $filename. Now, when we insert $filename into the open command, we are instructing the program to open pindata0.txt in the server's **data** folder and save the data in there. (If pindata0.txt does not exist, it is automatically created.)

We also open the data file **participation.txt** and record the fact that this user has completed another survey. Thus, when **pindemo2.pl** is activated later, there is one additional record for our user in this file, which will lead the value of $tasks to be one higher than it was previously.

The user is then told that his or her data were saved, and is presented with a button that allows him or her to return to the main menu. Notice that we pass $pin and $password along via hidden tags so that the user doesn't have to login again.

CUSTOMIZING THE CODE

In order to use this code for your own purposes, you'll need to do the following:

- Copy all of the code to separate blank documents and save them to your server's **cgi-bin** directory.
- In **pindemo2.pl**, alter the names of the surveys you want to appear in the menu. If you want to remain flexible, you can use labels such as "Section 1," "Section 2," and so on. Also, if you have a different number of sections than my four, modify accordingly.
- In **pindemo2.pl**, set the value of $numsurveys to equal the number of tasks or surveys that comprise your full study.
- Create each of your surveys or tasks as separate CGI scripts. Be sure to follow the example provided above in **pindemosurvey0.pl**. You'll need to read in $pin and $password from the CGI data packet, and you'll need to pass those values on via hidden tags. You'll also need to pass the survey or script number via a hidden tag.
- If you choose to use different names for your survey or task files (i.e., something other than **pindemosurvey1.pl**, for example), be sure to update the appropriate URLs in your scripts.
- Finally, you'll need to create a text file that contains all the valid PINs and passwords. You should model it after the example contents that we illustrated above. When people sign up for your study, you can send them a PIN number and the corresponding password. Alternatively, you can create a special script that allows users to create their own PIN and password.
- When you are ready to analyze the data, you'll need to import the survey text files into a spreadsheet program (see Chapter 5), sort the cases by PIN, and then merge the various files together while matching by PIN.

SUMMARY

In this chapter you have learned how to use Personal Identification Numbers (PINs) so that research participants can login to your site at any time and participate in multicomponent studies. These kinds of techniques can be useful in a variety of research contexts. For example, if you are conducting a longitudinal study in which you want participants to complete an attitude measure once a week over the course of several months, you could ask your participants to logon to your site once a week and fill out a questionnaire. The program would ensure that each participant's data were appropriately recorded. If you were conducting research that involved multiple components, you would want to give your participants the option to complete these components at different times. By using the methods discussed in this chapter, you can create a situation in which your user can complete one component at a time. Each time the user completes a component, the data are saved, and you, as the researcher, will not need to worry about losing data.

Here is a review of the Perl codes that were introduced in this chapter.

Perl commands	Function	Example
| ```
foreach $key (sort
($query-param)){
$value = $query->
param($key);
print INFO "$value,  ";
}
``` | This segment of code can be used to save data from the CGI pocket to a data file. In short, this code sorts the variable names in the data packet alphanumerically, then prints the value of each variable to the data file. Although this technique can be useful on occasion, the drawback is that it will not print values to the file if the user missed or omitted a questionnaire item. If a participant omits a response, an indication of that nonresponse is not set along with the CGI data packet. | ```
open(INFO,
">>c:\\data.txt");

foreach $key (sort
($query->param)){
$value = $query->
param($key);
print INFO "$value,  ";
}
print INFO "endline \n";
close(INFO);
``` |

Chapter 13

Measuring Response Times

Response times are often used to test hypotheses about mental processes. As we saw in Chapter 5, it is possible to obtain measures of time in online studies by requesting the time from the server's internal clock. By recording the time at which a CGI script sends a web page to a user's browser and the time a response to that page is submitted by the user, the total amount of time the user spent on a page can be calculated by simple subtraction.

How precise are timed measurements when recorded in this manner? As you might suspect, the measurement of response time to any one trial is fraught with problems. The value obtained will be influenced by a number of factors that have nothing to do with the psychological processes being investigated. For example, some users will be using computers with slower processors or slower modems. As a consequence, it may take them longer to load your page, and, hence, longer for them to respond to the stimuli. In addition, there are occasions when it simply takes a bit longer to load a page than it usually does. Even within the same measurement session, some trials might be slower to load than others. This delay may be due to how busy the server is at any one moment or random blips in Internet traffic that affect the overall rate of information transmission.

If we are conducting an experiment in which people are randomly assigned to conditions, it should be evident that the factors discussed above (e.g., browser type, computer speed, server activity, bandwidth constraints) are theoretically *uncorrelated* with the manipulation. If people are randomly assigned to conditions, there is no reason to expect speed problems to differ from one condition to the next. Of course, speed problems do affect the way we interpret the *absolute* response rates (i.e., speed errors *systematically increase* response times). However, we expect this systematic error to be constant across conditions. Therefore, by subtracting response times between conditions, the systematic errors are removed (i.e., a constant value minus the same value is zero), and differences between conditions will be more accurate.

Another issue worth considering is what unit of time is being measured. The smallest unit of time recorded by the server is the second. Thus, response time to any one trial is only precise to the nearest second. There are some research contexts, however, when the difference between conditions is expected to be at the level of milliseconds. As long as a sufficient number of people (or trials, in a within-subjects design) are used, this should not be a problem. Consider, for example, the fact that a sequence of measured times such as 2, 2, 3, and 2 seconds averages to 2.25 seconds. Although each measurement was recorded in seconds, the average of these measurements is in fractions of a second. By extension, the *difference* between conditions can be measured at the level of fractions of a second even when particular measurements are only in seconds.

A final point worth considering is that it can take anywhere from 0.5 to 2.5 seconds for a web page to fully load—even after all the relevant text is visible. As a consequence, the participant can often begin processing the stimulus before the information in the INPUT tags is fully loaded. If the user is ready to respond before the page is ready to be responded to, the user will have to wait before submitting his or her response. As a consequence, it is probably wise only to study response rates in experimental settings where it will take at least two seconds for the typical person to respond. For example, studies that require people to solve problems, retrieve complex information from memory, or read multiword stimuli would be appropriate for online reaction time research. Tasks that involve simple decisions that can be reached within a second (e.g., lexical decision tasks) would be inappropriate for online reaction time research using the methods reviewed here.

AN EXAMPLE: THE RECALL OF EMOTIONAL MEMORIES

To illustrate server-side time stamping techniques for measuring response times, let's create a simple experiment. In this demonstration, we'll ask participants to recall episodes from their past that were characterized by different emotions (i.e., happiness, loneliness, security, and anxiety). We'll vary the valence of the emotion (i.e., positive vs. negative) and see how much of a difference there is in the time it takes to recall positive vs. negative experiences from memory.

To exploit the time stamping feature of Perl, we need to use the multiple page techniques discussed in Chapter 9. Specifically, we'll need to stamp the time at which the HTML code was sent to the browser, as well as the time at which the next page's HTML code is sent to the browser (which occurs when the user submits a response). The difference between these times will be used as a measure of response time. I've created a flowchart (see Figure 13.1) that diagrams is process.

Let's begin with the simplest possible version of the study: One in which the order of stimuli is not randomized. Once we've outlined the basic techniques for recording response time, we'll build on the basic program to make it perform more complex tasks. Copy the following code to a blank document and save it as **rtdemo1.pl** in your server's **cgi-bin** folder. Also, run the program in your browser and try to get a feel for how the program operates.

<u>rtdemo1.pl</u>

```
#!C:/perl/bin/perl.exe
use CGI;
$query = new CGI;

$trials= 4;
$previoussec= $query->param('trialsec');
$previousmin= $query->param('trialmin');
$previoushour= $query->param('trialhour');

$rt00= $query->param('rt00');
$rt01= $query->param('rt01');
$rt02= $query->param('rt02');
$rt03= $query->param('rt03');
$trialnumber= $query->param('trialnumber');

#---------------------------
```

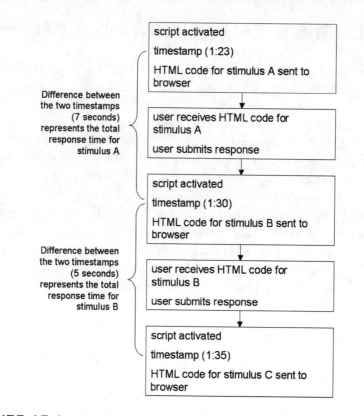

FIGURE 13.1. This chart illustrates the way in which response times are calculated in this chapter's scripts.

```
@varnum = ("00","01","02","03");
@stimuli= ("happy", "lonely", "secure", "anxious");

($sec,$min,$hour,$mday,$mon,$year,$wday,$yday,$isdst) =
    localtime(time);

#--------------------------

if($trialnumber != 0){
   $currenthour = $hour;
   $currentmin = $min;
   $currentsec = $sec;
   $rt= 0;
```

```
    # subtract seconds
    if($previoussec > $currentsec){
        $secdiff = ((60 + $currentsec) - $previoussec);
        $currentmin = $currentmin - 1;
    }

    if($previoussec <= $currentsec){
        $secdiff = $currentsec - $previoussec;
    }

    # subtract minutes
    if($previousmin > $currentmin){
        $mindiff = ((60 + $currentmin) - $previousmin);
        $currenthour = $currenthour - 1;
    }
    if($previousmin <= $currentmin){
        $mindiff = $currentmin - $previousmin;
    }

    # subtract hours
    if($previoushour > $currenthour){
        $hourdiff = ((24 + $currenthour) -
            $previoushour);
    }

    if($previoushour <= $hour){
        $hourdiff = $currenthour - $previoushour;
    }
    # convert difference to seconds
    $rt = (3600*$hourdiff)+(60*$mindiff)+($secdiff);

$temp = "rt" . $varnum[($trialnumber - 1)];
$$temp = $rt;
}
else{
    $trialnumber = 0;
}

print $query->header;
print $query->start_html(-title=>'Trials');
print "<FONT FACE = 'arial' SIZE = '2'>";

if($trialnumber >= 1){
```

```perl
    print "Time to recall on previous trial (seconds):
        $rt.<BR>";
}

#---------------------------

if($trialnumber < $trials ){

    print "<FORM ACTION = '/cgi-bin/rtdemo1.pl' METHOD
        = 'post'>";
    $stimulus= $stimuli[$trialnumber];
    print "<CENTER>Recall a time when you felt:
        <BR><BR>";
    print "<FONT FACE = 'arial' SIZE =
        '5'><B>$stimulus</B></FONT><BR><BR>";
    print "<I>Press the button when you have a specific
        experience in mind.</I><BR><BR>";
    print "<INPUT TYPE = 'submit' VALUE =
        'Ready'></CENTER>";

    $count= $trialnumber + 1;

    print "<INPUT TYPE = 'hidden' NAME = 'trialsec'
        VALUE = $sec>";
    print "<INPUT TYPE = 'hidden' NAME = 'trialmin'
        VALUE = $min>";
    print "<INPUT TYPE = 'hidden' NAME = 'trialhour'
        VALUE = $hour>";
    print "<INPUT TYPE = 'hidden' NAME = 'trialnumber'
        VALUE = $count>";
    print "<INPUT TYPE = 'hidden' NAME = 'rt00' VALUE
        = $rt00>";
    print "<INPUT TYPE = 'hidden' NAME = 'rt01' VALUE
        = $rt01>";
    print "<INPUT TYPE = 'hidden' NAME = 'rt02' VALUE
        = $rt02>";
    print "<INPUT TYPE = 'hidden' NAME = 'rt03' VALUE
        = $rt03>";

    print "</FORM>";
}

else{
    print "Thank you. You have finished all trials.
        <BR>";
```

```
    print "Here are your response times: <BR><BR>";
    print "$stimuli[0]  :  $rt00  seconds<BR>";
    print "$stimuli[1]  :  $rt01  seconds<BR>";
    print "$stimuli[2]  :  $rt02  seconds<BR>";
    print "$stimuli[3]  :  $rt03  seconds<BR>";
}

#---------------------------

print $query->end_html;
```

Let's dissect the script. As you can see from the FORM tag of the program rtdemo1.pl, this is a **recursive** script. In other words, each time the **Submit** button is clicked, the same script is activated again. Of course, each time the **Submit** button is pressed, the script is sending itself a CGI data packet, and the values within that packet will vary from one trial or "submission," to the next. As a consequence, the script will not behave the same way each time it is activated.

The first chunk of code is designed to read certain values from the submitted CGI data packet. If these values are empty, they are recorded as such. The first time the script is activated, there will be no CGI data packet, and all these variables will be empty.

The next section of the code creates some local variables that will be useful. The first line of code in this section creates an array, @varnum, that contains the placeholders for the various stimuli. The second line creates an array, @stimuli, that contains the actual stimuli: the kinds of emotional memories to be recalled. The third line of code in this section reads in the current time from the server's clock. The variables $hour, $min, and $sec will represent the hour, minute, and second at which the script was activated.

The next section of code is a series of nested if–else conditions. The first tests whether $trialnumber equals zero. $trialnumber is going to be a variable that we use to represent which trial the subject is on at any one point in the experiment. The first time through the script, $trialnumber does not have a value; it is empty. Thus, the first condition is not satisfied because the condition "$trialnumber does not equal zero" is false. As a consequence, the program executes the commands within the else braces. Within this section, the script simply explicitly assigns the value of $trialnumber to 0. Now, $trialnumber contains a real value (zero) and is no longer empty.

In the next segment of code, the script sets up some HTML parameters and prints the current stimulus to the user's browser. Notice that it is selecting, by using $trialnumber, the specific element of @stimuli to present to the user: $stimulus= $stimuli[$trialnumber]. Recall that $trialnumber currently equals 0; therefore, the script selects the 0th element of @stimuli, which is "happy." Thus, on this trial, the subject is asked to recall a happy memory.

Once the stimulus is presented, and the script is run again, the value of $trialnumber is incremented by one. (I have included an additional variable, $count, to update $trialnumber because in later scripts based on this one we will want to retain information about the current trial as well as getting ready for the next trial, which is what $trialnumber does.) Thus, the first time through the script, this value is updated from 0 to 1. Next, a number of hidden values are created. $trialhour, $trialmin, and $trialsec represent the time at which the script was activated. $trialnumber, which has been incremented by one, now represents the relevant trial number for the *next time* the script is activated. Finally, $rt00 through $rt03 represent the recorded reaction times for each trial. The first time through the script, these values are empty. Once the subject has recalled a happy memory and clicks the **Submit** button, these hidden values are passed in the CGI data packet.

Because the script is recursive, the same script is called again. This time, however, there are some values in the data packet, and the script assigns $trialnumer to equal 1. It also creates variables called $previoushour, $previousmin, and $previoussec and assigns those variables to equal the hour, minute, and second at which the data from the previous trial were processed by the server. We're going to use the difference between this time and the time at which the current script was activated (represented by $currenthour, $currentmin, and $currentsec) to estimate the response time for the *previous* trial.

When the if–else conditions are evaluated this time through, notice that $trialnumber equals 1. Because 1 is not equal to zero, the first condition is satisfied. Now the program is going to calculate the response time for the previous trial. I will not explain the details of how this code works, but essentially it functions to subtract the time (in hours, minutes, and seconds) the previous trial was activated from the time the current trial was activated. Because minutes and seconds are represented in a number system with a base of 60 instead of 10, the subtraction may look a bit odd at first. If the previous trial was initiated at 1:25:10 and the current trial was initiated at 1:25:30, the estimated reaction time will be 20 seconds.

Once the appropriate calculation is made, it is converted to seconds and assigned to the variable $rt ($rt = (3600*$hourdiff)+(60*$mindiff) +($secdiff);). Recall that we're calculating the response time to the previous trial, not the current trial. Thus, to assign $rt to the appropriate variable, we use the following commands:

```
$temp = "rt" . $varnum[($trialnumber - 1)];
$$temp = $rt;
```

In our example, $trialnumber currently equals 1. Thus, if we subtract 1 from it, the first command above extracts the 0th element of @varnum. This element equals "00." As a result, we end up appending the string "rt" to "00," creating the following string: rt00. We assign this string to the variable $temp. Thus, $temp equals rt00.

On the next line, we take the computed reaction time, $rt, and assign it to the variable $$temp. Because we have prefaced $temp with an extra dollar sign, the server reads $$temp as $rt00 (i.e., a dollar sign plus the value of $temp). In short, the server has taken the computed reaction time for the 0th trial and assigned it to the variable $rt00.

> **Note.** It is possible to append one string to another by using a period. For example, the following command $temp = "coffee " . "is good" will result in $temp being equal to coffee is good. Strings and variables can be appended in a similar manner. For example, $temp = "rt" . "$trialnumber" will result in $temp being equal to rt1, if $trialnumber is equal to "1." See Chapter 9 for more information.

Notice that the next time the script is activated, the value of $trialnumber will be 2, and the computed response time will be assigned to the variable label $rt01. This process continues until $trialnumber is equal to 4. At this point, the program skips to the else condition near the end of the script. This segment of code lists the response times for the four trials and thanks the user for his or her participation.

A MORE COMPLEX EXTENSION: SAVING THE DATA AND ANALYZING IT FOR THE PARTICIPANT

Now that we have a general script that can be used to collect response times from trial to trial (or page to page), let's expand the program to make it more useful. Specifically, let's take some of the skills we learned in Chapters 5 and 6 to save the data and analyze the data from the previous participants.

To accomplish this, we need to modify the commands within the final set of else braces. Therefore, replace the prior set of commands within the last set of else braces in **rtdemo1.pl** with those below. Save the revised document as **rtdemo2.pl** in your server's **cgi-bin** folder. Also replace print "<FORM ACTION = '/cgi-bin/rtdemorand2.pl' METHOD = 'post'>"; so that it recursively calls **rtdemo2.pl**. Try running the program to see how it behaves.

rtdemo2.pl

```
else{

    open(INFO,
      ">>$ENV{'DOCUMENT_ROOT'}/www/data/rtdemo.txt");
       print INFO "$mon/$mday/$year, $hour:$min:$sec, $ip, ";
       print INFO "$rt00, $rt01, $rt02, $rt03\n";
    close (INFO);

    open(INFO,
      "$ENV{'DOCUMENT_ROOT'}/www/data/rtdemo.txt");
       @data = <INFO>;
    close (INFO);

   print "Thank you. You have finished all trials.
     <BR>";
   print "Here are your response times: <BR><BR>";
   print "$stimuli[0]  :  $rt00  seconds<BR>";
   print "$stimuli[1]  :  $rt01  seconds<BR>";
   print "$stimuli[2]  :  $rt02  seconds<BR>";
   print "$stimuli[3]  :  $rt03  seconds<BR>";

   $mypos = ($rt00 + $rt02)/2;
   $myneg = ($rt01 + $rt03)/2;

   print "<BR>It took you $mypos seconds, on average,
```

to recall positive memories and $myneg seconds
to recall negative ones.

";

```
#---------------------------

    $sumpos = 0;
    $sumneg = 0;
    $n = 0;
       foreach $key (@data)
       {
           ($date,$time,$ip, $p01, $n01, $p02,
              $n02)=split(/,/,$key);
           $sumpos = $sumpos + (($p01 + $p02)/2);
           $sumneg = $sumneg + (($n01 + $n02)/2);
           $n = $n + 1;
       }
    $meanpos = sprintf("%.4f", ($sumpos/$n));
    $meanneg = sprintf("%.4f", ($sumneg/$n));

    print "On average, people in this sample have taken
       $meanpos seconds to recall positive memories and
       $meanneg to recall negative memories.<BR>";


}
```

In this version, the script computes an average response time for the two positively valenced trails (i.e., happy and secure) and the two negatively valenced trials (i.e., anxious and lonely). It does this with the following commands:

```
$mypos = ($rt00 + $rt02)/2;
$myneg = ($rt01 + $rt03)/2;
```

Notice that the program inserts these variables into the feedback that the user receives. That way, the user knows how he or she performed on the two kinds of trials.

There is also some code that calculates the average response time for positive and negative trials in the larger sample of participants. To do so, the script reads in the data from the text file **rtdemo.txt** in the **data** directory on your server and assigns them to the array @data. Using a for-each loop, the script assigns the values within each line of the data file to local variables (see Chapter 6 for more information on the foreach loop). As it runs through each line of the data file, it adds the average time for the two positive trials to a running sum called $sumpos. Similarly, it adds the average time for the two negative trials to a running total called $sumneg. Once the program has finished adding these values, it divides by the total number of subjects, $n, to obtain the mean response times across subjects to both kinds of trials. These means, rounded to four decimal places, are printed for the user.

BUILDING ON THE EXAMPLE: RANDOMIZING TRIAL ORDERS

In Chapter 7 we discussed the need to randomize the order in which trials are presented, and we discussed some techniques for doing so. Specifically, we reviewed a technique in which the stimuli order is determined in one script and passed onto a separate script that is responsible for presenting the trials. We'll adopt the same strategy here. Copy the two scripts below to blank documents and save them separately as **rtdemorand1.pl** and **rtdemorand2.pl** to your server's cgi-bin folder. Enter the URL for the first script and see how the program works.

rtdemorand1.pl

```
#!C:/perl/bin/perl.exe
use CGI;
$query = new CGI;

#---------------------------

   @trialorder = ("00", "01", "02", "03");
   srand;
   @new = ();
   while (@trialorder){
      push(@new, splice(@trialorder, rand @trialorder,1));
   }
   @trialorder= @new;

#---------------------------

print $query->header;
```

```
print $query->start_html(-title=>'Reaction Time Demo |
   Random Trials');

print "<FONT FACE = 'arial' SIZE = '2'>";
print "<FORM ACTION = '/cgi-bin/rtdemorand2.pl' METHOD
   = 'post'> ";

print $query->hidden('trialorder',@trialorder);

print "In this demonstration, you will be asked to
   recall different kinds of emotional experiences
   from your past.
      As soon as you're able to recall an experience
   that is characterized by the emotion printed in
   bold, click the button. The web page will then
   take you to the next recall trial. Please try to
   recall these experiences as quickly as
   possible.<BR><BR>";

print "<INPUT TYPE = 'submit' VALUE = 'Begin'>";
print "</FORM></FONT>";
print $query->end_html;
```

rtdemorand2.pl

```
#!C:/perl/bin/perl.exe
use CGI;
$query = new CGI;

#-------------------------

$trials= 4;
$previoussec= $query->param('trialsec');
$previousmin= $query->param('trialmin');
$previoushour= $query->param('trialhour');

$rt00= $query->param('rt00');
$rt01= $query->param('rt01');
$rt02= $query->param('rt02');
$rt03= $query->param('rt03');
$trialnumber= $query->param('trialnumber');
@trialorder= $query->param('trialorder');

#-------------------------

@varnum = ("00","01","02","03");
```

```perl
@stimuli= ("happy", "lonely", "secure", "anxious");

($sec,$min,$hour,$mday,$mon,$year,$wday,$yday,$isdst) =
   localtime(time);


#--------------------------

if($trialnumber != 0){
   $currenthour = $hour;
   $currentmin = $min;
   $currentsec = $sec;
   $rt= 0;
   $trialindex= $trialorder[$trialnumber];

   # subtract seconds
   if($previoussec > $currentsec){
      $secdiff = ((60 + $currentsec) - $previoussec);
      $currentmin = $currentmin - 1;
   }
   if($previoussec <= $currentsec){
      $secdiff = $currentsec - $previoussec;
   }

   # subtract minutes
   if($previousmin > $currentmin){
      $mindiff = ((60 + $currentmin) - $previousmin);
      $currenthour = $currenthour - 1;
   }
   if($previousmin <= $currentmin){
      $mindiff = $currentmin - $previousmin;
   }

   # subtract hours
   if($previoushour > $currenthour){
      $hourdiff = ((24 + $currenthour) - $previoushour);
   }
   if($previoushour <= $hour){
      $hourdiff = $currenthour - $previoushour;
   }

   # convert difference to seconds
   $rt = (3600*$hourdiff)+(60*$mindiff)+($secdiff);

   $temp = "rt" . $trialorder[($trialnumber - 1)];
   $$temp = $rt;
```

```
}
else{
   $trialnumber = 0;
   $trialindex= $trialorder[$trialnumber];
}

#---------------------------

print $query->header;
print $query->start_html(-title=>'Trials');
print "<FONT FACE = 'arial' SIZE = '2'>";

if($trialnumber >= 1){
   print "Time to recall on previous trial (seconds):
      $rt.<BR><BR>";
}

#---------------------------

if($trialnumber < $trials ){
   print "<FORM ACTION = '/cgi-bin/rtdemorand2.pl'
      METHOD = 'post'>";

   $stimulus= $stimuli[$trialindex];

   print "<CENTER>Recall a time when you felt:
      <BR><BR>";
   print "<FONT FACE = 'arial' SIZE =
      '5'><B>$stimulus</B></FONT><BR><BR>";
   print "<I>Press the button when you have a specific
      experience in mind.</I><BR><BR>";
   print "<INPUT TYPE = 'submit' VALUE =
      'Ready'></CENTER>";
   $count= $trialnumber + 1;
   print "<INPUT TYPE = 'hidden' NAME = 'trialsec'
      VALUE = $sec>";
   print "<INPUT TYPE = 'hidden' NAME = 'trialmin'
      VALUE = $min>";
   print "<INPUT TYPE = 'hidden' NAME = 'trialhour'
      VALUE = $hour>";
   print "<INPUT TYPE = 'hidden' NAME = 'trialnumber'
      VALUE = $count>";
   print "<INPUT TYPE = 'hidden' NAME = 'rt00' VALUE
      = $rt00>";
```

```perl
    print "<INPUT TYPE = 'hidden' NAME = 'rt01' VALUE
        = $rt01>";
    print "<INPUT TYPE = 'hidden' NAME = 'rt02' VALUE
        = $rt02>";
    print "<INPUT TYPE = 'hidden' NAME = 'rt03' VALUE
        = $rt03>";
    print $query->hidden('trialorder', @trialorder);
    print "</FORM>";
}

#---------------------------

else{

    open(INFO,
        ">>$ENV{'DOCUMENT_ROOT'}/www/data/rtdemo.txt");
        print INFO "$mon/$mday/$year, $hour:$min:$sec,
            $ip, ";
        print INFO "$rt00, $rt01, $rt02, $rt03\n";
    close (INFO);

    open(INFO,
        "$ENV{'DOCUMENT_ROOT'}/www/data/rtdemo.txt");
        @data = <INFO>;
    close (INFO);

    print "Thank you. You have finished all trials.
        <BR>";
    print "Here are your response times: <BR><BR>";
    print "$stimuli[0] : $rt00 seconds<BR>";
    print "$stimuli[1] : $rt01 seconds<BR>";
    print "$stimuli[2] : $rt02 seconds<BR>";
    print "$stimuli[3] : $rt03 seconds<BR>";

    $mypos = ($rt00 + $rt02)/2;
    $myneg = ($rt01 + $rt03)/2;

    print "<BR>It took you $mypos seconds, on average,
        to recall positive memories and $myneg seconds
        to recall negative ones.<BR><BR>";

#---------------------------

    $sumpos = 0;
    $sumneg = 0;
```

```perl
     $n = 0;
     foreach $key (@data)
     {
         ($date,$time,$ip, $p01, $n01, $p02,
            $n02)=split(/,/,$key);
         $sumpos = $sumpos + (($p01 + $p02)/2);
         $sumneg = $sumneg + (($n01 + $n02)/2);
         $n = $n + 1;
     }

  $meanpos = sprintf("%.4f", ($sumpos/$n));
  $meanneg = sprintf("%.4f", ($sumneg/$n));

  print "On average, people in this sample have taken
     $meanpos seconds to recall positive memories and
     $meanneg to recall negative memories.<BR>";

}

#---------------------------

print $query->end_html;
```

The first script welcomes the participant to the experiment, provides some brief instructions, and creates a random order in which the trials will be presented. This ordering is represented by the array @trialorder and is passed onto rtdemorand2.pl via a hidden tag when the **Submit** button is pressed.

The second script is organized much like the rtdemo2.pl script we studied before. However, it incorporates some features that allow it to present the stimuli in the random order set by @trialorder and save the response times in the appropriate manner. Here are some of the new features:

```perl
$trialindex= $trialorder[$trialnumber];
```

This line takes the current trial number (represented by $trialnumber) and uses that to index the specific trial to be used. Let's assume for a moment that @trialorder is equal to ("02," "03," "01," "00"). When $trialnumber is equal to 1, this code selects the 1st element of @trialorder, which is "03," and assigns that value to be equal to $trialindex. (Keep in mind that Perl begins indexing elements in an array using a value of 0. Thus, the 0th element of @trailorder is "02.")

The variable $trialindex will now be used to designate the index value for the stimuli to be presented.

```
$stimulus= $stimuli[$trialindex];
```

In our example, $trialindex equals 03. Thus, this line of code takes the 3rd element of @stimuli (i.e., "anxious") and assigns that string to be equal to $stimulus.

The other significant thing to note is in the following code:

```
$temp = "rt" . $trialorder[($trialnumber - 1)];
$$temp = $rt;
```

By using @trialorder here instead of @varnum (as we did in rtdemo1.pl and rtdemo2.pl), we are able to save the response time to the appropriate variable name, despite the fact that the trials are randomly ordered. If $trialnumber equals 1, then $trialnumber – 1 equals 0, and the 0th element of @trialorder (i.e., "02") is appended to "rt" and assigned to $temp. Thus, when we compute the reaction time, it will be the reaction time for the previous trial, which was designated by the 0th element of @trialorder.

SUMMARY

In this chapter you have learned how to measure the response times to web pages. By time stamping each submission, it is possible to estimate the time spent on a page by subtracting the time the submitted page was processed by the server from the time it was originally delivered to the user. Although this method only allows for a crude estimate of response time, it is possible to increase accuracy by averaging these estimates across trials or participants.

As is the case in non-Internet research, you will either want to include some practice trials for your participant before implementing the experimental trials or plan on deleting responses to the first few trials. Users will tend to take a bit longer to respond to the first few trials as they become accustomed to the interface.

Chapter 14

Additional Applications of Perl

Discussion Forums and Scored Tests

If you're a teacher, you've probably thought about using the techniques we've discussed in this book to supplement your courses. An obvious teaching application would be to create an online syllabus. By keeping your syllabus online, you can update it as needed (e.g., alert students to new reading assignments, post handouts, report answers to previous exams). Moreover, you can create hyperlinks to course notes, overheads, Microsoft PowerPoint (presentation) files, and other websites that might be relevant to the material you're covering.

You can, of course, accomplish all of these things without any knowledge of CGI scripting. However, the use of CGI scripting allows you to make the learning experience much more dynamic and interactive for you and your students. For example, you can easily adapt some of the skills acquired in previous chapters to create online quizzes and homework for students. Moreover, by exploiting the interactive nature of CGI scripting, you can create quizzes that provide students with feedback about their performance. In this chapter, I'll show you a script that can be used to create a generic quiz. To use it, all you'd need to do is supply your own questions and answers. Such quizzes can be used for teaching applications of course, but they can also be used in a variety of research contexts. So, although the example is a teacher's quiz, the chapter is useful regardless of whether you're a teacher.

We can also adapt the skills we've learned for reading and writing text files in order to create an online discussion forum. Online forums can be beneficial in a number of ways. In a teaching context, students can post questions and thoughts to the online forum, and you, as the instructor or teaching assistant, can post your replies. By having this exchange take place on the Web, you enable each student in your class to follow and contribute to the discussion, at their convenience. You may also want to use an online forum to initiate discussions of assigned readings. If you want to make sure that students are reading materials before a lecture, for example, you might ask them to post their reactions to the readings on the discussion forum before class. The online forum, of course, time stamps the submission so you know exactly when the comments were "turned in." Outside of a teaching context, a discussion forum may be used to host an online focus group. Focus groups are an excellent way of obtaining qualitative data from people, and, by hosting a focus group online, you can ensure an exact transcription of the dialogue.

The objective of this chapter is to illustrate how to create and use online quizzes and discussion forums. As I noted previously, we can create both of these by simply building on the "generic components" (e.g., creating HTML on the fly with CGI scripts, opening and writing to text files, creating questionnaires, using customized feedback) we have dealt with in previous chapters. We will, however, combine these components in novel ways to accomplish our tasks.

ONLINE DISCUSSION FORUM

The following set of scripts implements an online discussion forum. To use the forum, you'll need to copy each of the six CGI scripts below to separate blank documents and save each of them to your server's cgi-bin folder. After you've saved these scripts to the cgi-bin of your server, enter the URL for the forumdiscussion.pl script into the address bar of your browser. (To see a forum with a few postings go to this address on my website for this book: http://www.web-research-design.net/cgi-bin/forumdiscussion.pl.)

You should see a screen that looks like the one depicted in Figure 14.1 Since this is the first time you've used the program, there are no topics posted to your forum. Let's add one. Click on the button **Create a new topic**. This will automatically activate the script forumnewtopic.pl, which will take you to a new screen (see Figure 14.2).

Notice that there is a text box for a password. The default password for this forum is "stats." (I'll explain later how to change the password to one of your choosing.) Enter your name, the password, the subject of your post, and the actual message you would like to post. For the purposes of this demonstration and the screen shots that follow, I entered "Chris Fraley," "stats,"

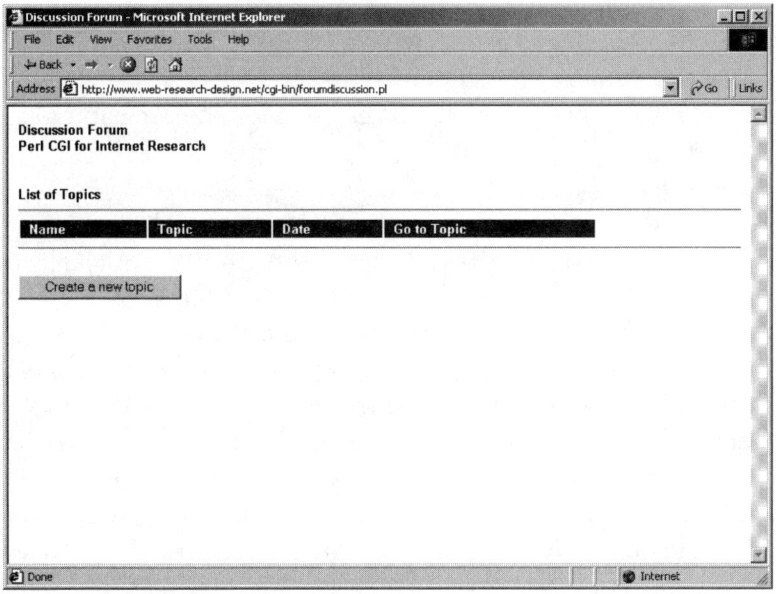

FIGURE 14.1. This page illustrates the main menu page of the discussion forum. The first time the discussion forum is accessed, there will be no active topics.

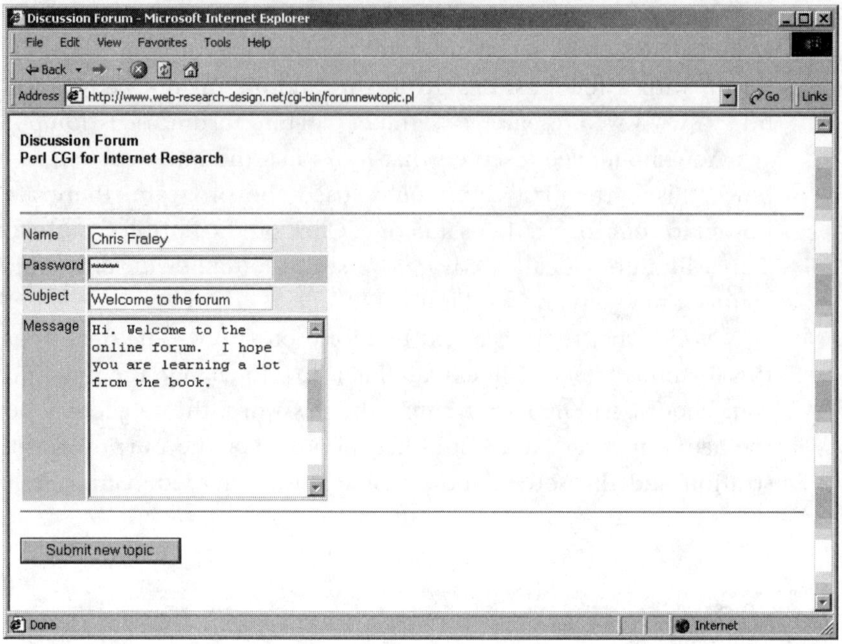

FIGURE 14.2. This page illustrates the interface for submitting a message to the forum.

"Welcome to the forum," and "Hi. Welcome to the online forum. I hope you are learning a lot from the book" in each of the respective text boxes. When finished, click on the **Submit new topic** button. Once you do so, and if the password was entered correctly, you should get a confirmation message. Click the button **Return to main page**. This will take you back to forumdiscussion. pl. However, now you should see an updated menu screen (see Figure 14.3).

Notice that the topic we just posted is listed on the forum. The author of the topic is listed as "Chris Fraley," the subject is "Welcome to the forum," and the date and time the topic was posted is listed. Post a few more topics, just so you can see how these pages work together. You should notice that each time you go back to forumdiscussion.pl, the list of forum topics is updated, and each entry is listed as a new row (see Figure 14.4).

Next to each topic listed there is a button labeled **Read**. Choose one of the topics and click on its corresponding **Read** button. Doing so will activate

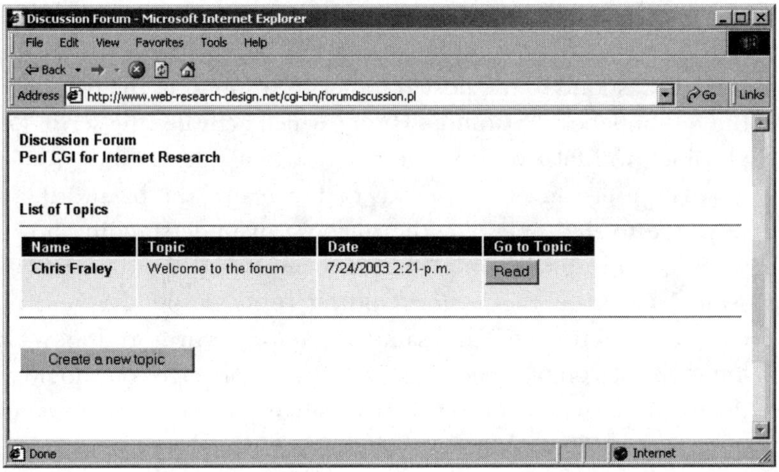

FIGURE 14.3. The menu page now includes the new topic we have submitted to the forum.

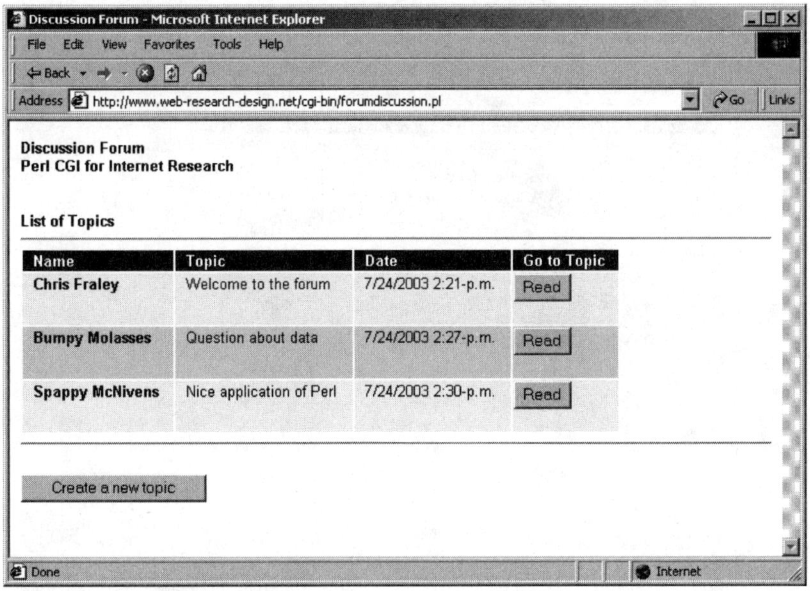

FIGURE 14.4. How the forum menu page looks when the forum has become more active.

the script forumgototopic.pl. This script displays the messages that corre-spond to the selected topic (see Figure 14.5). This script also allows forum users to respond to the posted topic. To respond to the posted topic, click on the button labeled **Submit a Reply**, which activates the script forumnewreply.pl, which will take you to a new page (see Figure 14.6).

The user can now enter his or her name, the password, and his or her response to the topic. For the purpose of understanding how these scripts work, go ahead and complete this form. Recall that the default password is "stats." Click on the button **Submit reply**. From the next page, you can choose to return to the same topic or return to the main page (i.e., forumdiscussion.pl). If you return to the topic page you should see your reply posted underneath the original message. Figure 14.5 shows an example of

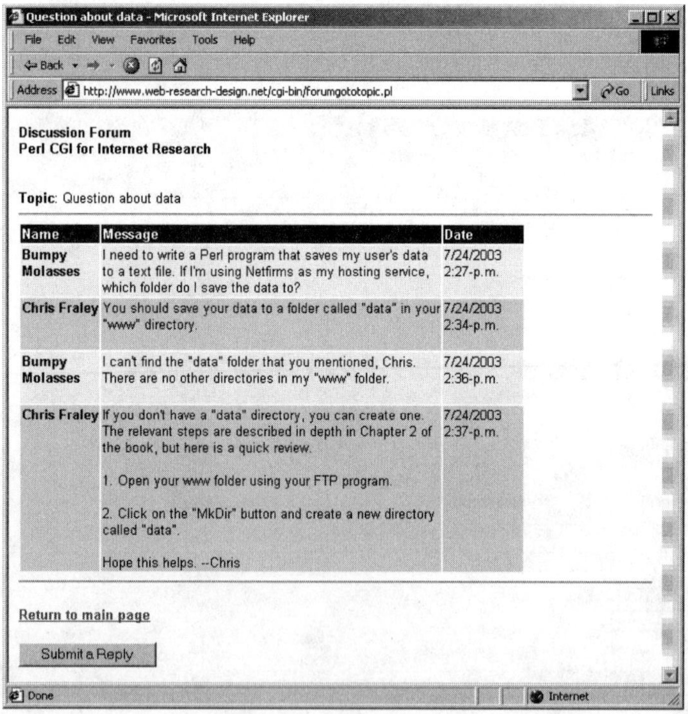

FIGURE 14.5. The interface for submitting a reply to an already existing topic.

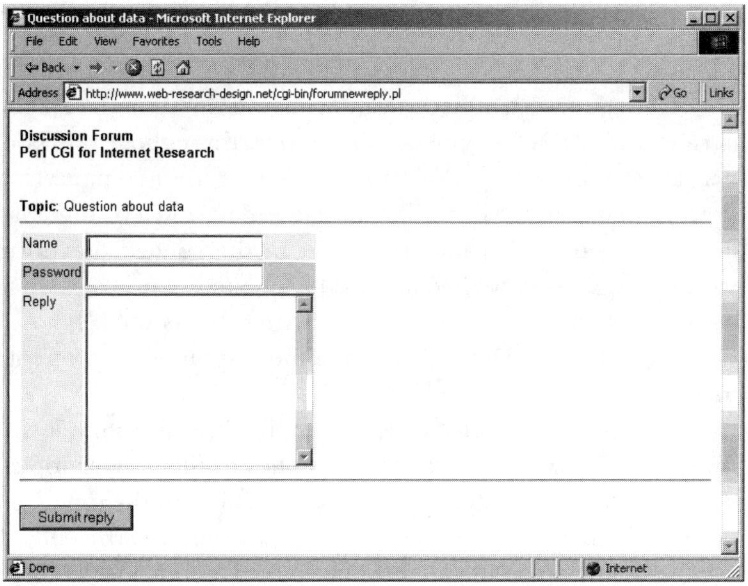

FIGURE 14.6. An example of a forum discussion on a specific topic.

what this page looks like after several replies have been posted under the topic called "Question about data."

Now that you have some hands-on experience using the forum, let's take a look at some of the text files that were created to store the data. Once you have a better sense of how the information in these files is organized, we'll be ready to dissect the CGI code and explain how the forum operates. Open the topics.txt file in your server's **data** directory. You should see a file that contains the various topics, the names of the authors of each topic, the actual messages, and the date and time they were posted. (This file was created automatically when you submitted a new topic. You don't need to create it by hand.) The text below represents a portion of the topics.txt data file created thus far based on my example.

```
Chris Fraley OOPHOIWelcome to the forum OOPHOIHi.
   Welcome to ...
Bumpy Molasses OOPHOIQuestion about data OOPHOII need
   to writ ...
```

```
Spappy McNivens OOPHOINice application of Perl
   OOPHOIHere is ...
```

Notice that each piece of information on a line is separated by the text string "OOPHOI." In previous examples throughout this book in which we used text files we separated the elements with a comma. In those cases we were working primarily with quantitative data and a comma was unlikely to be a part of the participant's response. In the context of a forum, however, a comma might very well be included in a person's message. To avoid this problem, one solution is to use a letter string that is unlikely to be typed by the user, such as OOPHOI, to separate the responses to different questions in a data file.

Now open the replys.txt file from the data directory. It is similar in structure to topics.txt and contains the replies to the various topics posted in the forum. The fact that the topics and the replies to the topics are stored in different files helps the server process the data more efficiently. If you find you have a highly active forum, it would be a good idea to modify the code so as to create different data files for each topic, which include that topic's responses.

The CGI Scripts and How They Work

Let's dissect the CGI scripts. I'll present each of the scripts below, along with a brief description of what they do and how they operate.

---

forumdiscussion.pl

```perl
#!C:/perl/bin/perl.exe
use CGI;
$query = new CGI;
$spacer= "OOPHOI";

open (INFO,
   "$ENV{'DOCUMENT_ROOT'}/www/data/topics.txt");
   @topics = <INFO>;
close (INFO);

print $query->header;
print $query->start_html(-title=>'Discussion Forum');
print "<FONT FACE = 'arial' SIZE = '2'>";
```

```perl
print "<B>Discussion Forum<BR>Perl CGI for Internet
   Research<BR></B><BR><BR>";

$temp= 1;

print "<B>List of Topics</B>";
print "<HR><TABLE WIDTH='80%'>";

print "<TR BGCOLOR='#330099'>
<TD><FONT FACE = 'arial' SIZE = '2'
   COLOR='white'><B>  Name  </B></TD>
<TD><FONT FACE = 'arial' SIZE = '2'
   COLOR='white'><B>  Topic  </B></TD>
<TD><FONT FACE = 'arial' SIZE = '2'
   COLOR='white'><B>  Date  </B></TD>
<TD><FONT FACE = 'arial' SIZE = '2'
   COLOR='white'><B>  Go to Topic  </B></TD>
</TR>";

foreach $key (@topics){
   if($temp == 1){
      print "<TR BGCOLOR='#F7F7F7' VALIGN='top'>";
      $temp= 2;
   }
   else{
      print "<TR BGCOLOR='#dedfdf' VALIGN='top'>";
      $temp= 1;
   }
   ($name, $subject, $message, $date1,
      $date2)=split(/$spacer/,$key);

   $temp2= "\"$subject\"";

   print "<TD><FONT FACE = 'arial' SIZE = '2'><B> 
      $name  </B></TD>
   <TD><FONT FACE = 'arial' SIZE = '2'>  $subject
       </TD>
   <TD> <FONT FACE = 'arial' SIZE = '2'>  $date1
      $date2  </TD>
   <TD><FORM ACTION='/cgi-bin/forumgototopic.pl'
      METHOD='post'>
   <INPUT TYPE='hidden' NAME='subjectselected'
      VALUE=$temp2>
   <INPUT TYPE='submit' VALUE='Read'></FORM></TD>
```

```
        </TR>";
    }

print "</TABLE><HR>";
print "<BR>";

print "<FORM ACTION='/cgi-bin/forumnewtopic.pl'
    METHOD='post'>";
print "<INPUT TYPE='submit' VALUE='Create a new
    topic'>";
print "</FORM>";

print $query->end_html;
```

The forumdiscussion.pl program acts as the opening, or main, page for the forum. When executed, this program will open a data base on the server (topics.txt) that contains all the topics that have been discussed on the forum and present them to the user. The user will be able to see each topic, the person who created it, and the date the topic was submitted. If the user wants to read the replies to a topic, he or she can click a button labeled **Read Replies**. Also, if the user wants to post a new topic, he or she can click on a button that will allow him or her to do so.

I'll review the code for this opening script in some depth because it contains the fundamental operations that are duplicated in the other scripts. The first three lines of code are the same three lines that open all the CGI scripts we've discussed in this book.

```
#!C:/perl/bin/perl.exe
use CGI;
$query = new CGI;
```

The next line creates a local variable called $spacer that will be assigned the text string "OOPHOI." We will use this value to separate the different pieces of information when saving information to a text file.

```
$spacer= "OOPHOI";
```

The next three lines of code open or create the text file topics.txt, the contents of which are read into the array @topics. Then the file is closed.

```
open (INFO,
  "$ENV{'DOCUMENT_ROOT'}/www/data/topics.txt");
@topics = <INFO>;
close (INFO);
```

The next lines of code instruct the server to send the user's browser the HTML code containing the title of the web page, "Discussion Forum."

```
print $query->header;
print $query->start_html(-title=>'Discussion Forum');
```

Next, we print something about the purpose of the forum. This will appear, in bold face type, at the top of the page. (You'll want to change this text to pertain to your forum.)

```
print "<B>Discussion Forum<BR>Perl CGI for Internet
  Research<BR></B><BR><BR>";
```

Next, we create a local variable named $temp and assign it a value of 1. The purpose of this variable will become clear in the next few sections.

```
$temp= 1;
```

Next, we instruct the server to create an HTML table. In the first row of the table, we're going to print the words "Name," "Topic," "Date," and "Go to Topic" in separate columns. Recall from our previous discussion of tables that we use the <TABLE> tag to begin a table, the <TR> and </TR> tags to start and end a row, and the <TD> and </TD> tags to start and end a column. Notice that we're specifying the background color of the row too by using the BGCOLOR attribute in the <TR> tag.

```
print "<B>List of Topics</B>";
print "<HR><TABLE WIDTH='80%'>";

print "<TR BGCOLOR='330066'>
<TD><FONT FACE = 'arial' SIZE = '2'
  COLOR='white'><B>  Name  </B></TD>
<TD><FONT FACE = 'arial' SIZE = '2'
  COLOR='white'><B>  Topic  </B></TD>
<TD><FONT FACE = 'arial' SIZE = '2'
  COLOR='white'><B>  Date  </B></TD>
```

```
<TD><FONT FACE = 'arial' SIZE = '2'
  COLOR='white'><B>  Go to Topic  </B></TD>
</TR>";
```

How will we get the background color for each row of the table to alternate between a lighter and darker gray? Before the for-each loop begins, the local variable $temp is set to 1. Once the for-each loop begins, an if–else condition sets the background color to #F7F7F7 (a very light gray; see Chapter 3 on hexadecimal color codes) if $temp equals 1. The first time through the loop then, $temp equals 1. Therefore, the background color is set to a light gray and $temp is changed to equal 2. The next time through the loop, the server will skip through the first condition because $temp is no longer equal to 1. Instead, it executes the commands in the else portion of the condition, setting the color to a darker gray (#dedfdf) and changing $temp back to 1. $temp equaling 1 again, the next time through the loop the first condition will be met, and the server will print the row with a light gray background. In short, each time the server cycles through the loop, it changes the value of $temp either from 1 to 2 or from 2 to 1, allowing it to alternate the colors of each row.

```
if($temp == 1){
   print "<TR BGCOLOR='#F7F7F7' VALIGN='top'>";
   $temp= 2;
}
else{
   print "<TR BGCOLOR='#dedfdf' VALIGN='top'>";
   $temp= 1;
}
```

Our next task is to take each line of data from @topics (i.e., the array that contains the information in the data file topics.txt), parse it into separate variables, and print the pertinent information to the web page. To do this, we create a for-each loop. The foreach command instructs the server to sort through each line of data in @topics. We're going to split each line of information into five variables (i.e., $name, $subject, $message, $date1, and $date2). Notice that we're *not* splitting the information on the basis of commas as we've done in previous examples. In this case, we're splitting the information on the basis of the occurrence of $spacer in the data file, which is "OOPHOI."

```
foreach $key (@topics){
  ($name, $subject, $message, $date1,
    $date2)=split(/$spacer/,$key);
  $temp2= "\"$subject\"";

  print "<TD><FONT FACE = 'arial' SIZE = '2'><B> 
    $name  </B></TD>
  <TD><FONT FACE = 'arial' SIZE = '2'>  $subject
     </TD>
  <TD> <FONT FACE = 'arial' SIZE = '2'>  $date1
    $date2  </TD>
  <TD><FORM ACTION='\cgi-bin\forumgototopic.pl'
    METHOD='post'>
  <INPUT TYPE='hidden' NAME='subjectselected'
    VALUE=$temp2>
  <INPUT TYPE='submit' VALUE='Read'></FORM></TD>
  </TR>";
}
```

Upon extracting these variables for one line of data, we print all but the $message variables to the different columns of our table in the order in which they were parsed. Finally, we create a form (<FORM...>), a hidden value, a **Submit** button, and close the form (</FORM>). This process continues until each row of data from @topics has been processed.

Recall that when the user clicks on one **Read** button at the end of each of these rows, a script is activated (forumgototopic.pl) that presents the topic and its corresponding replies. To ensure that the script knows which topic to present, we include the topic itself in the hidden tag created in the code above. To accomplish this, we've created a local variable called $temp2. We allow $temp2 to equal the value of $subject—the title or subject of the topic. Because the subject may be a complex phrase containing spaces, it is important to place quotes around the phrase. We can do this with the \" symbol (i.e., a slash followed by the quotes). If we did not place quotation marks around $subject, the hidden value tag would incorrectly parse the information. For example, if $subject were equal to How do I solve this problem? and we used the following command:

```
<INPUT TYPE='hidden' NAME='subjectselected'
  VALUE=$subject>
```

The user's browser would interpret it as

```
<INPUT TYPE='hidden' NAME='subjectselected' VALUE=How
  do I solve this problem?>
```

The browser would interpret the VALUE of this tag as being equal to "How" and ignore the rest of the text since these words do not correspond to any legitimate attributes of the tag. By placing quotes around the value of $subject, however, the browser correctly sees something like the following:

```
<INPUT TYPE='hidden' NAME='subjectselected' VALUE='How
  do I solve this problem?'>
```

Now the entire subject phrase is passed along as the VALUE of this hidden tag.

> **Note.** This is the first time in this book where we've used multiple forms on a single HTML page. Notice that doing so allows us to create multiple buttons that activate different scripts (or the same script with different hidden values).

Once the loop is complete, we close the table using the `</TABLE>` tag and create a new form. This form will contain its own **Submit** button that enables the user to create a new topic for the forum. Clicking this button activates forumnewtopic.pl.

```
print "</TABLE><HR>";
print "<BR>";
print "<FORM ACTION='/cgi-bin/forumnewtopic.pl'
  METHOD='post'>";
print "<INPUT TYPE='submit' VALUE='Create a new
  topic'>";
print "</FORM>";
print $query->end_html;
```

Going back, though, when the user selects a topic by clicking the **Read** button, the **forumgototopic.pl** script is activated. Let's study this script.

forumgototopic.pl

```
#!C:/perl/bin/perl.exe
use CGI;
$query = new CGI;
```

```perl
$subjectselected= $query->param('subjectselected');
$spacer= "OOPHOI";

open (INFO,
   "$ENV{'DOCUMENT_ROOT'}/www/data/topics.txt");
   @topics = <INFO>;
close (INFO);

open (INFO,
   "$ENV{'DOCUMENT_ROOT'}/www/data/replys.txt");
   @replys = <INFO>;
close (INFO);

$temp=1;

print $query->header;
print $query->start_html(-title=>$subjectselected);
print "<FONT FACE = 'arial' SIZE = '2'>";

print "<B>Discussion Forum<BR>Perl CGI for Internet
   Research<BR></B><BR><BR>";

print "<B>Topic</B>: $subjectselected<BR>";

print "<HR><TABLE WIDTH='80%'>";

print "<TR BGCOLOR='#330099' VALIGN='top'>
<TD VALIGN='top'><FONT FACE = 'arial' SIZE = '2'
   COLOR='white'><B>Name  </B></TD>
<TD VALIGN='top'><FONT FACE = 'arial' SIZE = '2'
   COLOR='white'><B>Message  </B></TD>
<TD VALIGN='top'><FONT FACE = 'arial' SIZE = '2'
   COLOR='white'><B>Date  </B></TD>
</TR>";

foreach $key (@topics){

   ($name, $subject, $message, $date1,
      $date2)=split(/$spacer/,$key);

   if($subject eq $subjectselected){

      if($temp == 1){
         print "<TR BGCOLOR='#F7F7F7' VALIGN='top'>";
         $temp= 2;
```

```perl
      }
      else{
         print "<TR BGCOLOR='#dedfdf' VALIGN='top'>";
         $temp= 1;
      }

   print "<TD VALIGN='top'>
   <FONT FACE = 'arial' SIZE = '2'>
   <B>$name   <BR> </B></TD>
   <TD VALIGN='top'> <FONT FACE = 'arial' SIZE =
      '2'>$message</TD>
   <TD VALIGN='top'> <FONT FACE = 'arial' SIZE =
      '2'>$date1 $date2 </TD></TR>";
   }
}

foreach $key (@replys){
   ($name, $subject, $message, $date1,
      $date2)=split(/$spacer/,$key);
   if($subject eq $subjectselected){
      if($temp == 1){
         print "<TR BGCOLOR='#F7F7F7' VALIGN='top'>";
         $temp= 2;
      }
   else{
      print "<TR BGCOLOR='#dedfdf' VALIGN='top'>";
      $temp= 1;
      }
   print "<TD VALIGN='top'>
   <FONT FACE = 'arial' SIZE = '2'>
   <B>$name   <BR> </B></TD>
   <TD VALIGN='top'> <FONT FACE = 'arial' SIZE =
      '2'>$message</TD>
   <TD VALIGN='top'> <FONT FACE = 'arial' SIZE =
      '2'>$date1 $date2 </TD></TR>";
   }
}

print "</TABLE>";
print "<HR><BR><A HREF='/cgi-bin/forumdiscussion.pl'>
   <B>Return to main page</B></A><BR>";
$temp2= "\"$subjectselected\"";
```

```
print "<FORM ACTION='/cgi-bin/forumnewreply.pl'
  METHOD='post'>";
print "<INPUT TYPE='hidden' NAME='date1'
  VALUE=$date1>";
print "<INPUT TYPE='hidden' NAME='date2'
  VALUE=$date2>";
print "<INPUT TYPE='hidden' NAME='subjectselected'
  VALUE=$temp2>";
print "<INPUT TYPE='submit' VALUE='Submit a Reply'>";
print "</FORM>";

print $query->end_html;
```

The operations in this script should be fairly evident given what we've covered so far; therefore, I'll restrict my comments to the basic functions of these operations. First, the server extracts some of the data submitted and assigns these values to local variables. One of the key pieces of information in the CGI packet is the subjectselected value. This value contains the topic the user selected, passed along in a hidden tag.

Next, the script opens the topics.txt data file and assigns the information within to the local array @topics. It also opens a file called replys.txt in the data folder on the server. This file contains the replies to the various topics. It assigns the information in this file to the local array @replys.

Using a for-each loop, the server cycles through each line of @topics. When it locates the line in which $subject is equal to $subjectselected, it prints the corresponding message (as well as the author, date, and time). When this loop is complete, it begins another for-each loop to detect the presence of replies to the current topic in @replies. When it finds lines to which the $subject variable is equal to $subjectselected, it prints the corresponding response, as well as the author of the response and the date and time it was submitted.

The last parts of the script provide a link back to the main page and a way for the user to add a reply to the messages posted on the current page. Specifically, it creates a form that activates a script named forumnewreply.pl when the **Submit** button is pressed. Moreover, some pertinent information (i.e., the topic of interest) is passed to the forumnewreply.pl script via hidden tags.

Here is the forumnewreply.pl script. This script is responsible for providing the user with a way to reply to a posted topic.

forumnewreply.pl

```perl
#!C:/perl/bin/perl.exe
use CGI;
$query = new CGI;
$subjectselected= $query->param('subjectselected');

($sec,$min,$hour,$mday,$mon,$year,$wday,$yday,$isdst) =
    localtime(time);
    $year = 1900 + $year;
    $mon= $mon+1;
    $ampm = "a.m.";
    if($hour > 12){
        $hour= $hour - 12;
        $ampm = "p.m.";
    }
    $date1= "$mon/$mday/$year";
    $date2= "$hour:$min" . "-" . "$ampm";

print $query->header;
print $query->start_html(-title=>$subjectselected);
print "<FONT FACE = 'arial' SIZE = '2'>";

print "<B>Discussion Forum<BR>Perl CGI for Internet
    Research<BR></B><BR><BR>";

print "<FORM ACTION='/cgi-bin/forumsavereply.pl'
    METHOD='post'>";

print "<B>Topic</B>: $subjectselected<BR>";

print "<HR><TABLE>
<TR BGCOLOR='#F7F7F7'>
<TD VALIGN='top'><FONT FACE = 'arial' SIZE = '2'>
    Name </TD>
<TD> <INPUT TYPE='textbox' NAME='name' MAXLENGTH='30'
    SIZE='25'></TD>
</TR>

<TR BGCOLOR='#dedfdf'>
<TD VALIGN='top'><FONT FACE = 'arial' SIZE = '2'>
    Password </TD>
<TD> <INPUT TYPE='password' NAME='password'
    MAXLENGTH='30' SIZE='25'></TD>
</TR>

<TR BGCOLOR='#F7F7F7'>
```

```
<TD VALIGN='top'><FONT FACE = 'arial' SIZE = '2'>
   Reply </TD>
<TD> <TEXTAREA NAME='message' COLS=25 ROWS=10
   WRAP='virtual'></TEXTAREA></TD></TR>";
print "</TABLE><HR>";
print "<BR>";

$temp2= "\"$subjectselected\"";

print "<INPUT TYPE='hidden' NAME='date1'
   VALUE=$date1>";
print "<INPUT TYPE='hidden' NAME='date2'
   VALUE=$date2>";
print "<INPUT TYPE='hidden' NAME='subjectselected'
   VALUE=$temp2>";
print "<INPUT TYPE='submit' VALUE='Submit reply'>";
print "</FORM>";

print $query->end_html;
```

This script creates several text boxes for the user to enter his or her name, the password, and the text of his or her message or response. When the user is finished, he or she clicks the **Submit reply** button, which activates forumsavereply.pl. Several hidden values are passed to this script: the date ($date1), the time ($date2), and the topic itself ($temp2—the value of subjectselected with quotations around it).

Notice that we've processed the date information slightly. As you'll recall from Chapter 5, the year 2002 is encoded as 102. To translate this value to the appropriate year, we simply add 1900 to $year. Also, the value of the month ($mon) is encoded such that January is equal to zero and December is equal to 11. To "correct" this start-with-zero coding, we add 1 to the value of $mon. Finally, instead of reporting the hour in 24-hour time, we have an if–then conditional that subtracts 12 from the value of $hour when $hour is greater than 12. Thus, if the time is 15 hours, this change will set the hour to 3 (i.e., 3 o'clock).

The next script, forumsavereply.pl, is responsible for taking the user's reply and saving it to the reply.txt data file. Here is the script:

forumsavereply.pl

```
#!C:/perl/bin/perl.exe
use CGI;
```

```perl
$query = new CGI;

$name= $query->param('name');
$subjectselected= $query->param('subjectselected');
$message= $query->param('message');
$date1= $query->param('date1');
$date2= $query->param('date2');
$password= $query->param('password');
$spacer= "OOPHOI";

print $query->header;
print $query->start_html(-title=>'Discussion Forum');

if($password eq "stats"){
   $message =~ s/\n/<BR>/g;
   $message =~ s/\r/ /g;

   open (INFO,
     ">>$ENV{'DOCUMENT_ROOT'}/www/data/replys.txt");
     print INFO "$name$spacer";
     print INFO "$subjectselected$spacer";
     print INFO "$message$spacer";
     print INFO "$date1$spacer";
     print INFO "$date2\n";
   close (INFO);

   print "<FONT FACE = 'arial' SIZE = '2'>";
   print "<B>Discussion Forum<BR>Perl CGI for Internet
     Research<BR></B><BR><BR>";

   print "Your reply has been saved.<BR>";
   print "<FORM ACTION='/cgi-bin/forumgototopic.pl'
     METHOD='post'>";

   $temp2= "\"$subjectselected\"";

   print "<INPUT TYPE='hidden' NAME='subjectselected'
     VALUE=$temp2>";
   print "<INPUT TYPE='submit' VALUE='Return to topic'>
     ";
   print "</FORM>";
   print "<FORM ACTION='/cgi-bin/forumdiscussion.pl'
     METHOD='post'>";
   print "<INPUT TYPE='submit' VALUE='Go to main
     page'>";
```

```
    print "</FORM>";
}
else{
    print "<FONT FACE = 'arial' SIZE = '2'>";
    print "<B>Discussion Forum<BR>";

    print "You entered an invalid password.<BR>
    If you think you have made an error, please use
        the <I>back</I> button on your browser and try
        again.";
}

print $query->end_html;
```

This script assigns some of the values in the CGI data packet to local variables. Next, it opens the text file **replys.txt** and prints those values to the file. Notice that we're separating each value with the $spacer variable, which is equal to OOPHOI. After we've printed the last piece of information to the file, we use the symbol for a new line (\n) and close the data file. The script then tells the user that the response was saved successfully, and provides him or her with the option of returning, back to the individual topic page or to the main page.

It is important to note that this script only saves the data if the password has been entered correctly. The program checks for this with the following command:

```
if($password eq "stats"){
```

If the value of $password is "stats," the program executes the commands that save the response. If the value of $password is something else, the program executes the commands in the else braces. Specifically, it tells the user that he or she entered the incorrect password.

> **Note.** If you want to change the password to one of your choosing, replace the word *stats* with the new password. You'll need to make this change in this script, as well as the script called **forumsavetopic.pl** discussed later. If you want to have separate passwords for each user, you can adapt the code used in Chapter 12.

> **Note.** The following line of code probably looks alien: $message =~ s/\n/
/g. This command takes each occurrence of a carriage return in $message and replaces it with an HTML line break. Without this substitution, the carriage return would be encoded as a real carriage return in the data file and would create errors in the way the data are processed.

The next two scripts work the same way as the previous two. The first, forumnewtopic.pl, is activated when the user wants to create a new topic at the main page. This script accepts the new information and passes it on to forumsavetopic.pl, using hidden tags. forumsavetopic.pl checks the password and saves the new topic to topics.txt. Finally, it gives the user the option to return to the main page.

forumnewtopic.pl

```perl
#!C:/perl/bin/perl.exe
use CGI;
$query = new CGI;

($sec,$min,$hour,$mday,$mon,$year,$wday,$yday,$isdst) =
    localtime(time);
    $year = 1900 + $year;
    $mon= $mon+1;
    $ampm = "a.m.";
    if($hour > 12){
        $hour= $hour - 12;
        $ampm = "p.m.";
    }
    $date1= "$mon/$mday/$year";
    $date2= "$hour:$min" . "-" . "$ampm";

print $query->header;
print $query->start_html(-title=>'Discussion Forum');

print "<FONT FACE = 'arial' SIZE = '2'>";

print "<B>Discussion Forum<BR>Perl CGI for Internet
    Research<BR></B><BR><BR>";

print "<FORM ACTION='/cgi-bin/forumsavetopic.pl'
    METHOD='post'>";

print "<HR><TABLE>
```

```
<TR BGCOLOR='#F7F7F7'>
<TD VALIGN='top'><FONT FACE = 'arial' SIZE = '2'>
  Name </TD>
<TD> <INPUT TYPE='textbox' NAME='name' MAXLENGTH='30'
  SIZE='25'></TD>
</TR>

<TR BGCOLOR='#dedfdf'>
<TD VALIGN='top'><FONT FACE = 'arial' SIZE = '2'>
  Password </TD>
<TD> <INPUT TYPE='password' NAME='password'
  MAXLENGTH='30' SIZE='25'></TD>
</TR>

<TR BGCOLOR='#F7F7F7'>
<TD VALIGN='top'><FONT FACE = 'arial' SIZE = '2'>
  Subject </TD>
<TD> <INPUT TYPE='textbox' NAME='subject'
  MAXLENGTH='30' SIZE='25'></TD>
</TR>

<TR BGCOLOR='#dedfdf'>
<TD VALIGN='top'><FONT FACE = 'arial' SIZE = '2'>
  Message </TD>
<TD> <TEXTAREA NAME='message' COLS=25 ROWS=10
  WRAP='virtual'></TEXTAREA></TD></TR>";
print "</TABLE><HR>";
print "<BR>";

print "<INPUT TYPE='hidden' NAME='date1'
  VALUE=$date1>";
print "<INPUT TYPE='hidden' NAME='date2'
  VALUE=$date2>";
print "<INPUT TYPE='submit' VALUE='Submit new
  topic'>";
print "</FORM>";

print $query->end_html;
```

forumsavetopic.pl

```
#!C:/perl/bin/perl.exe
use CGI;
$query = new CGI;
```

```perl
$name= $query->param('name');
$subject= $query->param('subject');
$message= $query->param('message');
$date1= $query->param('date1');
$date2= $query->param('date2');
$password= $query->param('password');
$spacer= "OOPHOI";

print $query->header;
print $query->start_html(-title=>'Discussion Board');

if($password eq "stats"){
   $message =~ s/\n/<BR>/g;
   $message =~ s/\r/ /g;

   open (INFO,
      ">>$ENV{'DOCUMENT_ROOT'}/www/data/topics.txt");
      print INFO "$name $spacer";
      print INFO "$subject $spacer";
      print INFO "$message $spacer";
      print INFO "$date1 $spacer";
      print INFO "$date2\n";
   close (INFO);

   print "<FONT FACE = 'arial' SIZE = '2'>";

   print "<B>Discussion Forum<BR>Perl CGI for Internet
      Research<BR></B><BR><BR>";

   print "Your message has been saved.<BR>";

   print "<FORM ACTION='/cgi-bin/forumdiscussion.pl'
      METHOD='post'>";
   print "<INPUT TYPE='submit' VALUE='Return to main
      page'>";
   print "</FORM>";
}

else{
   print "<FONT FACE = 'arial' SIZE = '2'>";
   print "<B>Discussion Forum<BR>Perl CGI for Internet
      Research<BR></B><BR><BR>";

   print "You entered an invalid password.<BR>
   If you think you have made an error, please use
```

```
        the <I>back</I> button on your browser and try
        again.";
}

print $query->end_html;
```

Summary of the Online Forum Programs

The online forum is implemented with six scripts, each responsible for a unique function. Here is a simple overview of each script and the tasks for which it is responsible.

- **forumdiscussion.pl**   This script creates the main page. It reads all the existing topics from the topics.txt data file and prints them to a web page in an organized manner. It also provides the user with the option of reading any of the existing topics or creating a new topic.
- **forumgototopic.pl**   Is activated when the user hits the **Read** submit button. It prints the messages that are pertinent to that topic and also provides the user with the option of adding his or her own message to the page.
- **forumnewreply.pl**   This script is activated when the user chooses to add a reply to a discussion within a topic. The page provides input boxes for the user's name, the forum password, and the reply message itself.
- **forumsavereply.pl**   Is activated when the user submits a new reply to a topic. This script checks to see if the password is valid. If it is valid, the script saves the reply to the replys.txt data file. If not, the script tells the user that the password was incorrect.
- **forumnewtopic.pl**   This script is activated when the user chooses, on the main page, to create a new topic. It provides input boxes for the user's name, the forum password, the topic, and the new subject message itself.
- **forumsavetopic.pl**   Is activated when the user submits a new topic. This script checks to see if the password is valid. If it is, the script saves the topic to the topics.txt data file. If not, the script tells the user that the password was incorrect.

The scripts are sufficiently generic for you to modify and use for your own purposes. To do so, you'll need to replace the sections of each script that read, "Discussion Forum, Perl CGI for Internet Research," with the appropriate information for your purposes. Also, if you want to change the password, you'll need to modify the default password, "stats," in the if–then portions of the forumsavereply.pl and forumsavetopic.pl scripts. If you want to remove the password option completely, delete the portions of the scripts that involve passwords. This includes the password text box in the forumnewreply.pl and forumnewtopic.pl scripts and the if–else conditions in the forumsavereply.pl and forumsavetopic.pl scripts.

> **Note.** If you want to create multiple forums for different purposes (e.g., one for a discussion group, one for a class), you will need to do one of two things. One option is to create separate directories for each purpose and save copies of the scripts in each directory. Another option is to incorporate a new name for each script file name. For example, if you were teaching Psych 101 and Psych 242 you could create two copies of the forumdiscussion.pl file, one called psych101discussion.pl and the other called psych242discussion.pl. (Similarly, you could rename the other scripts in the same fashion.) You would need to alter the names of the files in the various FORM elements of the scripts that are responsible for activating other scripts. You would also need separate topics.txt and replys.txt files in a similar manner.

ONLINE QUIZZES

One way to help students prepare for exams is to give them periodic quizzes. Unfortunately, administering quizzes in class can take away valuable lecture and discussion time. Moreover, grading paper-and-pencil quizzes can take an extraordinary amount of time. Online quizzes can solve both of these problems. Students can complete online quizzes without your having to use class time to administer them. And, by using CGI scripting, the server automatically grades the quizzes. It saves you time and can give your students instant feedback.

The generic script presented below uses a multiple-choice format to quiz students. Once the student has answered each question, the script grades the quiz, tells the student the correct answers, and allows him or her to retake the quiz. This particular quiz script randomly selects a subset of questions from a larger group of questions. Thus, each time the student retakes the quiz, he or she will get a randomly selected set of questions that may or may not overlap with those seen before.

Copy the script to a blank document and save it as onlinequiz.pl in your cgi-bin directory. Type the URL into your browser address bar, and take the quiz. This particular quiz tests your knowledge of HTML and CGI programming in Perl. I have only included five questions, from which the script selects three to display for each time through the quiz. Figure 14.7 shows a screen shot of the quiz in action.

Once you answer the questions and click on the **Grade my quiz** button, you'll receive feedback on your answers. (Figure 14.8 shows the feedback).

Here is the script. Below I'll explain the code.

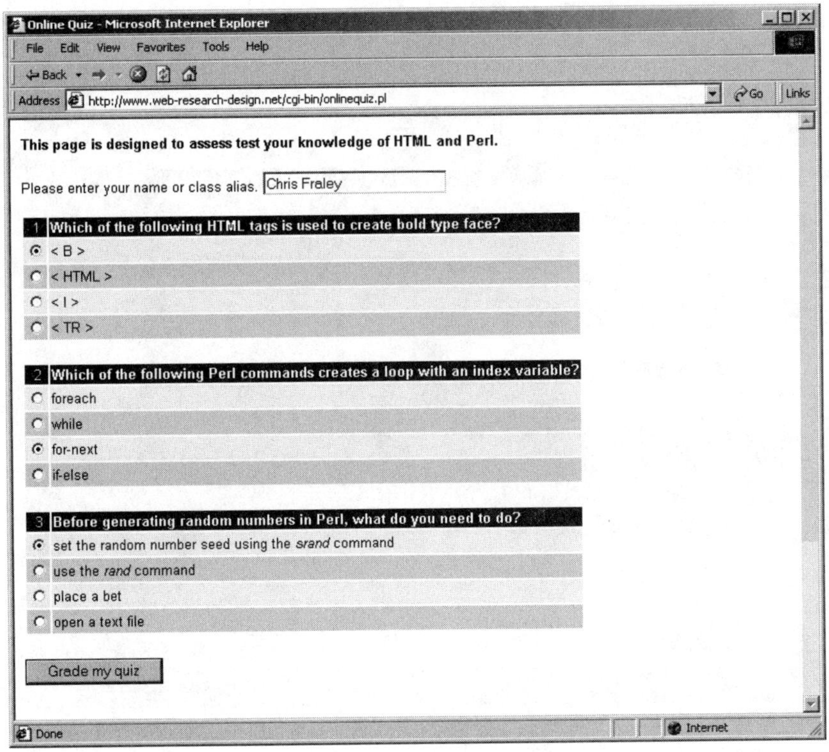

FIGURE 14.7. An example of an online quiz.

onlinequiz.pl

```
#!C:/perl/bin/perl.exe
use CGI;
$query = new CGI;

#---------------------------------------------

$n= 3;
```

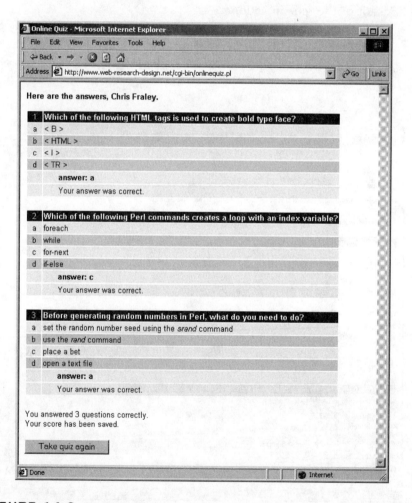

FIGURE 14.8. The Perl script automatically grades the quiz and tells the user how he or she performed.

```
$total= 5;

$q0= "Which of the following HTML tags is used to
   create bold type face?";
$q0a= "\< B \> ";
$q0b= "\< HTML \> ";
$q0c= "\< I \> ";
$q0d= "\< TR \> ";

$q1= "Which of the following HTML tags is used to
   create a new row in an HTML table?";
$q1a= "\< B \> ";
$q1b= "\< HTML \> ";
$q1c= "\< I \> ";
$q1d= "\< TR \> ";

$q2= "Which of the following Perl commands creates a
   loop with an index variable?";
$q2a= "foreach";
$q2b= "while";
$q2c= "for-next";
$q2d= "if-else";

$q3= "Which of the following <I>tricks</I> can be
   used to overcome statelessness?";
$q3a= "Use an if-else condition";
$q3b= "There is no adequate way of handling the
   statelessness problem";
$q3c= "Use JavaScript";
$q3d= "Use hidden tags to pass submitted data to new
   pages";

$q4= "Before generating random numbers in Perl, what
   do you need to do?";
$q4a= "set the random number seed using the
   <I>srand</I> command";
$q4b= "use the <I>rand</I> command";
$q4c= "place a bet";
$q4d= "open a text file";

@answers= ("a", "d", "c", "d", "a");

#------------------------------------------------

$r0= $query->param('r0');
```

```perl
$r1= $query->param('r1');
$r2= $query->param('r2');
$r3= $query->param('r3');
$r4= $query->param('r4');

$alias= $query->param('alias');

#--------------------------------------------------

$timethrough= $query->param('timethrough');
@varlist= $query->param('varlist');

#--------------------------------------------------

if($timethrough != 1){

   @varlist= ("0", "1", "2", "3", "4");
   srand;
   @new = ();
   while (@varlist){
      push(@new, splice(@varlist, rand @varlist,1));
   }
   @varlist= @new;

   print $query->header;
   print $query->start_html(-title=>'Online Quiz');
   print "<FONT FACE = 'arial' SIZE = '2'>";
   print "<B>This page is designed to assess test your
      knowledge of HTML and Perl.</B><BR> <BR>";
   print "<FORM ACTION = '/cgi-bin/onlinequiz.pl'
      METHOD = 'post'> ";

   print "Please enter your name or class alias. ";
   print "<INPUT TYPE='textbox' NAME='alias'
      MAXLENGTH='35' SIZE='25'><BR><BR>";

   print "<TABLE>";
   for($i = 0; $i <= ($n - 1); ++$i){
      $questionnumber= $i + 1;
      $question= "q" . $varlist[$i];
      $optiona= $question . "a";
      $optionb= $question . "b";
      $optionc= $question . "c";
      $optiond= $question . "d";
```

```perl
       print  "<TR BGCOLOR='#330099'><TD><FONT
         FACE='arial'  COLOR='white' SIZE='2'>   
         $questionnumber</TD><TD><FONT FACE='arial'
         COLOR='white' SIZE='2'><B> $$question
         </B></FONT></TD></TR>
       <TR BGCOLOR= '#F7F7F7'> <TD><INPUT TYPE = 'radio'
         NAME = r$varlist[$i] VALUE = 'a'></TD><TD>
         <FONT FACE='arial' SIZE='2'> $$optiona
         </TD></TR>
       <TR BGCOLOR= '#dedfdf'> <TD><INPUT TYPE = 'radio'
         NAME = r$varlist[$i] VALUE = 'b'></TD><TD>
         <FONT FACE='arial' SIZE='2'> $$optionb
         </TD></TR>
       <TR BGCOLOR= '#F7F7F7'> <TD><INPUT TYPE = 'radio'
         NAME = r$varlist[$i] VALUE = 'c'></TD><TD>
         <FONT FACE='arial' SIZE='2'> $$optionc
         </TD></TR>
       <TR BGCOLOR= '#dedfdf'> <TD><INPUT TYPE = 'radio'
         NAME = r$varlist[$i] VALUE = 'd'></TD><TD>
         <FONT FACE='arial' SIZE='2'> $$optiond
         </TD></TR>
       <TR BGCOLOR= 'white'><TD>   </TD><TD>  
         </TD></TR>";
   }
   print "</TABLE>";

   print $query->hidden('varlist',@varlist);
   print "<INPUT TYPE='hidden' NAME='timethrough'
     VALUE='1'>";
   print "<INPUT TYPE = 'submit' VALUE = 'Grade my
     quiz'>";
   print "<BR></FORM></FONT>";
   print $query->end_html;
}

#----------------------------------------------------

else{
   $numbercorrect= 0;
   ($sec,$min,$hour,$mday,$mon,$year,$wday,$yday,$isdst)
     = localtime(time);
   $year = 1900 + $year;
   $mon= $mon+1;
   $date= "$mon/$mday/$year/$hour/$min";
```

```
print $query->header;
print $query->start_html(-title=>'Online Quiz');
print "<FONT FACE = 'arial' SIZE = '2'>";
print "<B>Here are the answers,
  $alias.</B><BR><BR>";

print"<TABLE>";
for($i = 0; $i <= ($n - 1); ++$i){
  $correctanswer= $answers[$varlist[$i]];
  $questionnumber= $i + 1;
  $question= "q" . $varlist[$i];
  $optiona= $question . "a";
  $optionb= $question . "b";
  $optionc= $question . "c";
  $optiond= $question . "d";

  print "<TR BGCOLOR='#330099'><TD><FONT
    FACE='arial' COLOR='white' SIZE='2'>  
    $questionnumber  </TD><TD><FONT
    FACE='arial' COLOR='white' SIZE='2'><B>
    $$question </B></FONT></TD></TR>
  <TR BGCOLOR= '#F7F7F7'><TD><FONT FACE='arial'
    SIZE='2'>   a   </TD><TD><FONT
    FACE='arial' SIZE='2'> $$optiona </TD></TR>
  <TR BGCOLOR= '#dedfdf'><TD><FONT FACE='arial'
    SIZE='2'>   b   </TD><TD><FONT
    FACE='arial' SIZE='2'> $$optionb </TD></TR>
  <TR BGCOLOR= '#F7F7F7'><TD><FONT FACE='arial'
    SIZE='2'>   c   </TD><TD><FONT
    FACE='arial' SIZE='2'> $$optionc </TD></TR>
  <TR BGCOLOR= '#dedfdf'><TD><FONT FACE='arial'
    SIZE='2'>   d   </TD><TD><FONT
    FACE='arial' SIZE='2'> $$optiond </TD></TR>
  <TR BGCOLOR= '#F7F7F7'><TD>   </TD><TD><FONT
    FACE='arial' SIZE='2'><B>      
    answer: $correctanswer</B></TD></TR>
  <TR BGCOLOR= '#F7F7F7'><TD>   </TD><TD><FONT
    FACE='arial' SIZE='2'>";

  $answerselected= "r" . $varlist[$i];
  if($correctanswer eq $$answerselected){
    print "       Your answer was
      correct.";
    $numbercorrect = $numbercorrect + 1;
    }
```

```
      else{
      print "       Your answer,
         $$answerselected, was incorrect.";
      }
    print "<TR BGCOLOR= 'white'><TD>   </TD><TD>
         </TD></TR>";
    }
    print "</TABLE>";

#-------------------------------

    open(INFO,
       ">>$ENV{'DOCUMENT_ROOT'}/www/data/onlinequiz.txt")
       ;
       print INFO "$alias OOPHOI $date OOPHOI
          $numbercorrect\n";
    close(INFO);

#-------------------------------

    print "You answered $numbercorrect questions
       correctly.<BR>";
    print "Your score has been saved.<BR>";
    print "<FORM ACTION = '/cgi-bin/onlinequiz.pl'
       METHOD = 'post'> ";
    print "<INPUT TYPE='hidden' NAME='timethrough'
       VALUE='0'>";
    print "<INPUT TYPE='hidden' NAME='alias'
       VALUE=$alias >";
    print "<INPUT TYPE = 'submit' VALUE = 'Take quiz
       again'>";
    print $query->end_html;
  }
```

The basic code is the same as that used earlier when we randomized the order of self-esteem questions (see Chapter 6). There are, however, three things worth noting here. First, for the purposes of compacting the code, two major functions have been forced into a single script. The two key functions are (1) presenting the test questions and (2) grading the responses. We could have created two scripts to handle these functions. The server can determine what to do according to if–else commands. The first time the script is activated, the CGI packet value destined for $timethrough does not exist because no data packet was submitted to the server. Thus, when the server reaches the following command: `if ($timethrough != 1) {}` (read as "If the value of $timethrough does not equal 1, then execute the commands within braces"), it processes the commands within braces because $timethrough does not equal 1. The commands within these braces instruct the server to randomize the order of the questions and present a subset of those questions to the user (`for ($1 = 0; $i < = ($n - 1); ++$i)`). A **Grade my quiz Submit** button is also created. Pressing this button reactivates the script, and sends all the responses (and hidden values) to the server.

Notice that one of the hidden values changes $timethrough to 1. Thus, the second time through the script, it assigns the value of 1 to the local variable $timethrough. Now, when the server reaches the `if ($timethrough != 1) {}` command, it skips through the commands in braces and executes the commands within the else braces. These commands print the questions again, grades the questions, and shows the correct answers. A **Take quiz again Submit** button is created. When this button is clicked, $timethrough is changed to 0 and encoded as a hidden value, and the script is reactivated. The user receives a new random subset of the questions.

To customize the script for your own purposes, there are a few things you'll need to do:

- Substitute your questions (and response options) for the ones in the script. If you want to make more than five questions, add the new questions and increment the $a1 names accordingly. If you use more than 10 questions, you'll need to change the numbers to two digits (e.g., change 0 to 00, 1 to 01, 2 to 02).
- The variable $total represents the total number of questions available. If you have more than five questions in your question bank, you'll need to change this value. The variable $n indicates the number of questions to be asked. Set this value to the number of questions you want to be asked at any one time. If you want all the questions in your item bank to be presented, set $n equal to the total number of questions ($total).
- In the array called @answers, enter the correct answer to each question in the order in which you've placed the questions in the script.

There are many ways this program could be expanded or modified to make it suit your purposes. For example, you might want to keep a record of which students have taken the quiz, how many times they took it, and their performance. To do this, you would need to (1) create an input box for the student to enter his or her name and (2) a section of code that opens a text file, saves the student's name and the number of questions answered correctly, and closes the file. If you wanted to omit telling the students the correct answers, you could eliminate the portion of the code that prints the answers.

Chapter 15

Wrapping It Up

My objective in this book has been to teach you a number of generic skills that can be combined to create a wide variety of research studies. By now, I hope that you have a reasonable grasp of some of the techniques.

Although my primary focus has been on teaching you *how* to create online studies, there are a number of issues pertaining to online research that we've yet to discuss. These include troubleshooting techniques, methods for getting your site known, ethical concerns, server maintenance, security, sampling issues, participant dropout, data quality control, and web design. In this final chapter, I'll discuss each of these matters. A whole book could be devoted to several of these topics in their own right; I'll refer you to noteworthy resources whenever appropriate.

TROUBLESHOOTING

It can be an incredibly frustrating experience when you're trying to get your code to work and, for some unknown reason, it isn't working the way you want it to, or worse, it isn't working at all. Here is a list of some things to keep in mind when you're trying to troubleshoot or "debug" your CGI scripts.

1. Make sure that each line of commands in your Perl script ends with a semicolon. This is one of the most common errors; so, no matter how silly it sounds, be sure to double-check problematic code to ensure that there is a semicolon at the end of each line.

2. Make sure that each opening brace ({) has a corresponding closing brace (}). Also, double check to see that each HTML tag requiring a closing tag has one and that each opening quote has a closing quote. A common mistake is to create a web form using the <FORM> tag but omit the </FORM> tag.

3. Make sure that the Perl/CGI scripts are in your server's cgi-bin directory and that your HTML files are in your server's Public HTML directory. If you're using a professional web hosting service, make sure that new files and the most recent updates of files have been transferred to your server. You will receive different error messages if the requested file is missing versus if the requested file has an error.

4. It is easy to use double quotes in the wrong context. Keep in mind that you should not use double quotes in a CGI script except in the places we've discussed. It is okay—and necessary—to use double quotes in the following command: print "This coffee tastes good"; However, if you wanted to print a sentence that contains quotations around a phrase or word, it is better to use single quotes: print "This 'coffee' tastes good";.

5. One frustrating thing about programming in Perl is that, if a Perl script has a syntax error, the script often will not run at all and you may see a message similar to that shown in Figure 15.1. Such a message, unfortunately, doesn't help you identify the source of the problem. One way to hone in on the problem is by using a debugging feature called "fatalsToBrowser." To use this feature, insert the line use CGI::Carp qw(fatalsToBrowser); immediately after the she-bang! line. Now, when server attempts to run the script, errors that prevent it from running will be printed directly to your browser window. This will allow you to see what kinds of problems may exist in your code.

To see an example of how this works, consider the buggy program below:

```
#!C:/perl/bin/perl.exe
use CGI::Carp qw(fatalsToBrowser);
use CGI;
$query = new CGI;
```

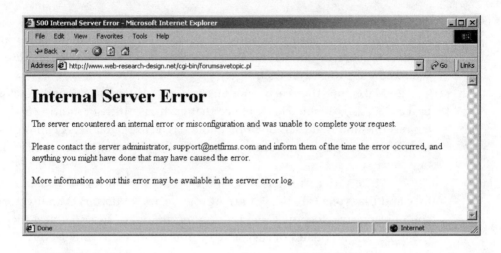

FIGURE 15.1. An error message I received when I made mistakes in my programs.

```
print $query->header;
print $query->start_html(-title=>'Error Free Web Page');

$sum = 0;
print "The value of sum is now $sum <BR>";

for($i=0; $i<10;++$i){
   $sum = $sum + 10;
   print "The value of sum is now $sum <BR>;
}

print $query->end_html;
```

If you study this code carefully, you'll notice that there is a quotation mark missing in the following line: `print "The value of sum is now $sum <BR>;`. When this script is executed, the browser window will produce the output illustrated in Figure 15.2. Notice that the server has told us that it had trouble finding an expected quotation mark on line 14. This information will make it easier to debug our program.

6. Sometimes a script will be fine as far as its syntax is concerned (i.e., Perl will not complain), but it may not be working quite the way you expect it

to. There are at least two useful ways to debug a script in this circumstance. One approach is to "comment out" parts of your script in a systematic and strategic manner. As we discussed in Chapter 10, you can use the pound sign to temporarily instruct Perl to ignore an instruction: #print "This coffee tastes good"; By temporarily "commenting out" a line in this manner, you can see if the script runs correctly without it. If you still have a problem after commenting out a line or a block of lines, you know that the problem exists elsewhere. At that point, you can simply remove the pound signs without having to retype the lines again.

Another helpful technique is to print the values of your local variables at different points in the script to ensure that the values of the variables are updating as expected. Let's assume, for example, that you had a variable, $sum, that is supposed to be incremented each time it passes through a loop. You could insert the following line within your loop in order to see the value of $sum each time it passes through the loop: print "The value of sum is $sum";

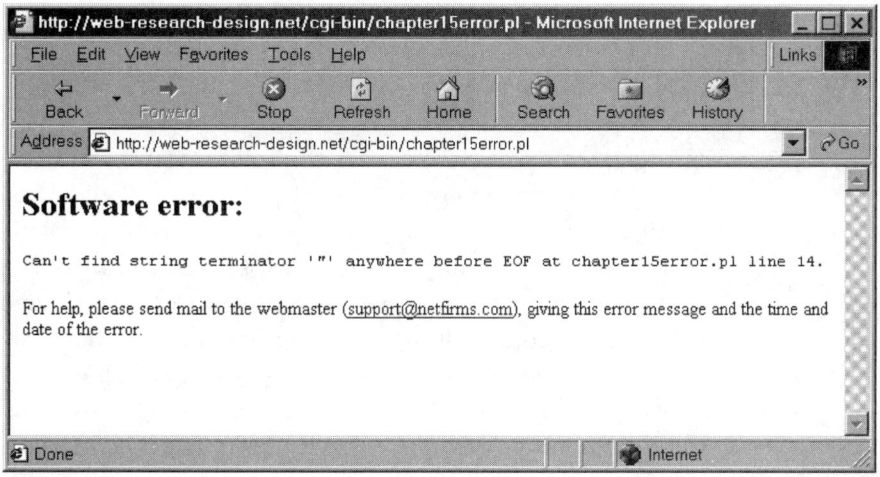

FIGURE 15.2. When the fatalsToBrowser command is used, any errors that prevent your Perl script from running will be sent to the browser window.

7. Perl is "case sensitive." This means that the program treats lowercase letters differently from uppercase letters. As a consequence, the variable $sum is not the same as $Sum. When a variable isn't behaving the way you expect, check to see that the case of letters in variable names does not differ. (As a side note, URL addresses are *not* case sensitive. As a result, http://www.web-research-design.net/ is the same as http://www.Web-Research-Design.net/.)

8. If you have done everything discussed above and you're still unable to get your script to work, you might want to try downloading a Perl editor that will check the syntax for your Perl scripts. The DZSoft Perl Editor is a Perl editor that many people find useful. You can download free evaluation copies of the program at the DZSoft website: http://www.dzsoft.com/dzperl.htm. In order for the program to work correctly, you'll need to download a copy of Perl (see Chapter 2 on downloading ActiveState Perl). In addition to providing the kind of code and syntax coloring that 1st Page uses, the DZSoft editor will allow you to "run" your code on your own computer, outside of the website environment, and it will tell you where coding problems may exist. This function can be quite useful, but it doesn't always work reliably with complex code (e.g., code that involves writing to files and reading from files).

GETTING YOUR SITE KNOWN

If you want to recruit participants over the Internet, there are several, cost-free ways to make your site known to people. First, you should create a home page for your lab (see Chapter 3) that has an up-to-date list of the various online studies that are currently available at your web lab. By having a stable page (i.e., one that will be around even as your specific studies come and go), it is more likely that people will find your site. Second, you should register the URL for the home page of your website with popular search engines. Yahoo!, for example, organizes its searches by subject areas. You'll want to register the URL for your site under the area that is most relevant to your site (see http://docs.yahoo.com/info/suggest/).

Third, you'll want to make sure the title of your home page closely matches the kinds of keywords someone might use if they were interested in participating in online research. A good title might contain the phrase, "free online research in psychology."

Several years ago, most search engines relied heavily on the keywords contained in META tags—hidden HTML tags that contain descriptors for the page, but no actual HTML code per se. Unfortunately, many web designers abused these tags and would include everything that you can imagine—regardless of relevance—within the tags just to ensure that their pages would rise to the top. As a consequence, many search engines stopped weighting META tags heavily in ranking the results of a search. Nonetheless, you can still use these tags to help get your page listed. Here are some examples of META tags, which if used are placed right under the TITLE tag in the HTML code for a page:

```
<META NAME='description' CONTENT='Learn more about
    your personality with this free, online personality
    test'>
<META NAME='keywords' CONTENT='personality, online,
    quiz, free, self-scoring'>
```

Google, one of the most effective search engines, ranks pages largely by their "centrality" in the WWW. That is, the more pages that exist with links to page x, the more likely it is that page x will be ranked highly in a search. Google uses this information, coupled with powerful pattern matching algorithms that analyze the content of a page, to rank web pages. Therefore, you should consider asking colleagues to create links to your home page on their sites.

If people find your site truly useful (i.e., if your experiments provide informative feedback for your users, are relatively brief, and new research appears frequently), it may happen that people will create links to your site without an explicit request. One thing you should keep in mind is that search engines do not necessarily index your CGI scripts; they typically index only the pages in your Public HTML directory. Thus, make sure that your home page is a standard HTML document that resides in your server's Public HTML directory.

Many scientific organizations in psychology have web pages that list URLs to online research. For example, the American Psychological Society has a page maintained by John Krantz that keeps an up-to-date listing of online studies (http://psych.hanover.edu/Research/exponnet.html). You might want to visit this site and submit the URL for your page. You should also visit the Web Experimental Psychology Lab (http://www.psychologie.

unizh.ch/genpsy/Ulf/Lab/WebExpPsyLab.html), run by Ulf-Dietrich Reips, one of the pioneers in online psychological research.

ETHICS

If you plan to use the Internet to conduct research you'll need to create a way to obtain informed consent from your participants. This is done easily enough online. For any experiment you create, you'll need to design an opening page that, in addition to providing instructions for the study, provides a brief overview of what the research is about, and how long it will take to complete the study. You should also include a **Submit** button that the user needs to press to begin the experiment. The button should have a caption that reads something like, "By clicking this button, I certify that I have read the above information and that I am 18 years of age or older." Figure 15.3 shows an example from one of the research studies in my web lab.

You'll also need IRB (Institutional Review Board) approval from your research institution before conducting human-subjects research over the Internet. At the University of Illinois at Chicago, getting IRB approval for Internet research is mostly a formality, for two reasons. The first is that Internet participation is fully voluntary; research subjects can withdraw, quite literally, from the research at any time. The second important factor is that we do not collect personal identifying information from our research subjects. In other words, we have no way of knowing from whom the data come. For my university, when our research violates these two conditions, we must submit more complex protocols to the IRB.

If a study needs to be deceptive in order to be effective, can that be done ethically in an online context? It isn't currently clear whether this is possible and I would strongly discourage you from implementing an online experiment that requires deception, for a few reasons. First, some social science disciplines already have a bad reputation for misleading research participants. Although some research suggests that participants do not mind mild forms of deception in laboratory experiments (Epley & Huff, 1998), it is easier to explain the nature of the deception in face-to-face debriefing sessions. Moreover, in an educational institution, where a lot of behavioral research is conducted, it is probably easier for participants to appreciate the benefits of

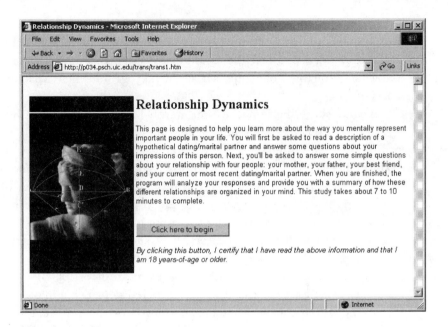

FIGURE 15.3. An example of an informed consent for an online study from my lab.

research and the need for deception in certain contexts. It isn't clear whether a nonstudent visiting your site is going to appreciate the fact that mild deception is sometimes necessary in order to get more truthful answers to certain questions. Finally, without a face-to-face debriefing, it can be difficult to ascertain how the deception has affected the subject. I would argue that it would be difficult to justify the use of deception in online research.

APACHE SERVER MAINTENANCE

If you chose to operate your own server, as opposed to using a professional web hosting service, you will need to *maintain* the server. Although the server requires very little attention or active maintenance, there are some things you'll need to keep an eye on. First, your Apache server will create log files that track the activity on your website. Each time someone accesses a page from your site, the server creates a record of when it happened, what page was accessed, and the IP address of the requesting computer. This information is appended to a text file called **access** that is ordinarily located in the following directory of your server: C:\Program Files\Apache Group\Apache2\logs\.

If your site is fairly active (i.e., if you have a number of files that get accessed in the course of a single experiment, or if you have a lot of people visiting your site), the access log will get large very quickly and will slow the performance of your server enormously. Whenever the access file has more than 10,000 entries, it is probably wise to turn off your server, delete the access log, then restart your server. The next time your site is accessed, a new access log will be created. (If you don't want to delete your access log, you can simply move it to a separate directory. I keep a separate directory of old access logs in case I ever need to refer to them.)

Your server also sends error messages to an error log file. It is wise to check this error log periodically to see if there is a problem in one or more of your web pages. If you can't get a page to work the way you want it to, you can often find a detailed description of where the program is breaking down in the error log. Like the access log, the size of this file can affect your server's performance. Be sure to delete or move the error log periodically to keep your server operating smoothly.

It should go without saying that it is always a good idea to create back ups of your web pages, Perl scripts, and data files. I try to make a habit of copying all my data files to a zip disk every two weeks.

SECURITY: PROTECTING YOUR SERVER

How do you prevent malicious programmers from hacking into your server and disrupting your research? There is no foolproof way to keep this from happening. One of the fundamental laws of the Universe, apparently, is that any system can be cracked, no matter how secure it may seem. There are, nonetheless, a number of things you can do to minimize the likelihood that less skilled hackers can obtain access to your server.

How can you tell whether someone is trying to hack your server? If you are using your own Apache server, you can check your server's error log. (If you're using a professional web hosting service, contact the service regarding access to error logs.) From time to time you'll notice odd error messages—messages that aren't as simple as "no semicolon at end of line 13." It might appear that someone was trying to access a file that they could not access (hence the recorded error message) or trying to run a program unsuccessfully from your computer.

Don't take these hacking attempts personally. There are many viruses in circulation that take over people's computers and send these malicious commands to IP addresses the computer has visited in the past. In other words, it probably is not the case that someone is sitting in a dim, smoke-filled room trying to break into *your* server. Most of the trouble stems from automated programs executed on helpless, virus infected computers.

If you notice repeated hacking attempts originating from the same IP address, you might want to incorporate some code into your programs that turns users at that IP address away. Recall from Chapter 5 that it is easy to determine the IP address of a computer that is calling one of your scripts. Before any of the substance of your script is executed, you could include a line that redirects the user to another website (or a page on your site that says something like "Access Denied") if his or her IP address is on your list of banned IP's:

```
$ip= $query->remote_addr();
if($ip =~ /135.234.543.23/){
    print $query->redirect("http://www.google.com");
}
```

There are a couple more things you can do to help protect yourself. First, it is wise to back up your files from time to time—just in case something goes horribly wrong. I try to back up everything (i.e., HTML files, scripts, and data) every two weeks simply by copying the contents of my key server files to a zip disk. Second, whenever your script accepts input from a user, strip that input of any information that is inappropriate or unwanted. For example, you can use the following command to remove carriage returns (which can easily mess up a text file) from a response called $value:

```
$value =~ s/\r//g;
```

One way for people to disrupt your server is by sending your CGI script data that does not originate from one of your web pages. In a typical application, you may send form data to a specific script for processing. A user of your web page can study the HTML code and determine the URL for the CGI script that is called when the **Submit** button is pressed. Then, he or she can write a script on his or her own server that passes data to your script. This unwanted data could taint the data that you are saving from your subjects or contain commands that are designed to hack into your system. Fortunately, there is a way to check to see whether the data are being submitted from your site. For example, the following CGI code extracts information about the "referrer"— the URL of the web page from which the user submitted the data—and sends the user elsewhere if that URL does not contain the URL for my website.

```
$ref= $query->referer();
if($ref !~ /web-research-design.net/){
   print $query->redirect("http://www.google.com");
}
```

To the best of my knowledge, no one has hacked into my Apache server successfully. I suspect that most programmers who try to hack into protected systems typically do so because they enjoy the challenge. If you were a major business or high-tech firm, you'd probably more likely be a target than if you were a graduate student in psychology. However, your naïveté may be another reason for hackers to try to take over your system. A hacker might want to take over your system and use it as a base for breaking into other systems. This might not interfere with your data collection per se, but it could pose a number of other problems. If you do suspect someone is trying to hack your system, you should contact your institution's or web hosting service's computer technical support immediately.

SECURITY: PROTECTING YOUR DATA

In this book we discussed some ways to save data from your participants to text files on your server. We have not discussed how to protect those text files from being viewed by other web users. If you are using Netfirms, you should be able to see the data files that we've been creating throughout this book by going to the appropriate directory: yourdomain/data/textfile.txt. Similarly, if you've setup your own Apache server, the text files can be viewed by going to the appropriate directory: yourdomain/web/data/textfile.txt.

To prevent web users from viewing or accessing your data files, you'll need to alter the permissions on those files. I'll explain how to do this separately for readers using a web hosting service, such as Netfirms, and for those with their own Apache server.

Professional Web Hosting Service. If you are using Netfirms or another web hosting service, you can use your FTP program to prevent people from viewing the data in your **data** folder.

1. Open an FTP connection to your server.

2. Click on the **data** directory within the **www** directory to highlight it. Don't open it; simply highlight it.

3. Using your mouse, right-click once on the folder. A new menu will appear. Select the **Properties** option. (In older versions of WS_FTP Pro, the option might be called **Permissions** or **Chmod**.)

4. Under the **Owner** options, make sure each box (i.e., **Read**, **Write**, **Execute**) is selected. For the **Group** and **Other** options, select the **Write** option and *deselect* the **Read** and **Execute** options. This will instruct the server to not allow anyone other than you to view the contents of the data folder (see Figure 15.4).

5. Press the **OK** button. If the program asks you if you would like to apply these new permissions to all the files in the folder, indicate **Yes**.

    Once you have completed these steps, no one will be able to view the files in your **data** folder by simply typing in the appropriate URL. You, however, will still be able to logon to your server using your FTP program and transfer the data files to your computer for analysis. Be careful not to alter the permissions for your **www** folder. You do want people to be able to view the contents of your **www** directory.

Your Own Apache Server. If you've set up your own Apache web server, you can use an alternative directory in which to store your data files. I would recommend creating a new directory in your **Apache2** folder called **data**. When you begin writing your own research scripts, replace the lines of code from the examples in this book that have the following form:

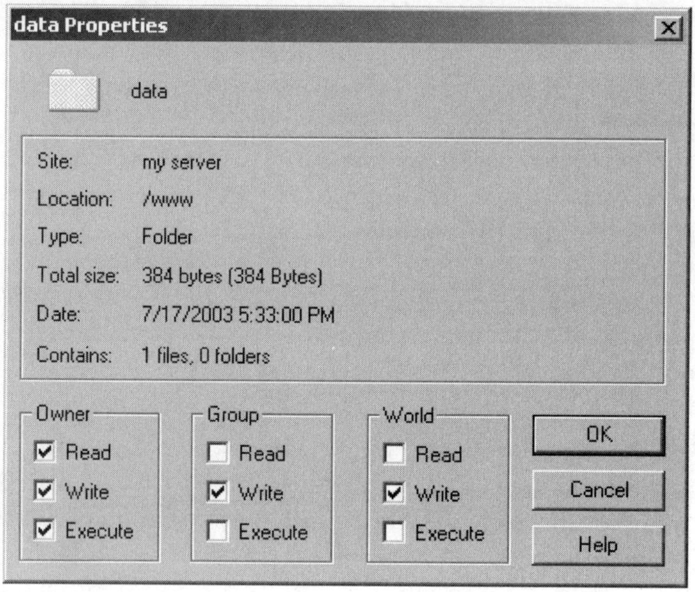

FIGURE 15.4. If you're using your FTP program to change the permissions on your server's **data** directory, make sure the boxes are selected/deselected in the way shown in this figure.

```
open (INFO,
    ">>$ENV{'DOCUMENT_ROOT'}/www/data/datafile.txt");
```

or

```
open (INFO,
    "$ENV{'DOCUMENT_ROOT'}/www/data/datafile.txt");
```

with the following:

```
open (INFO, ">>C:\\Program Files\Apache Group\Apache2\
    data\replys.txt");
```

or

```
open (INFO, "C:\\Program Files\Apache Group\Apache2\
    data\replys.txt");
```

Because the new **data** folder is no longer within your **Public HTML** folder (i.e., the **htdocs** directory), web users will not be able to view its contents. Your server will still be able to write data to files in this folder and you will still be able to access the contents of this folder in the same way you would access any other file on your computer (e.g., using the **My Computer** application).

SAMPLING ISSUES

To date, I've relied on the Internet largely as a way to collect data from research subjects that I haven't recruited *from* the Internet. I often use our department's student subject pool to recruit my participants, and then ask them to do the studies online. Participating online makes the process more interesting and convenient for my participants, and allows me to randomize questionnaire items easily, provide my subjects with customized feedback, and have the data stored and processed automatically. However, as I noted in the beginning chapter, one of the exciting prospects of Internet research is the ability to obtain research participants from anywhere.

Recruiting research subjects online, of course, raises many sampling concerns. What kind of sample are you likely to obtain by allowing anyone surfing the Web to participate in your study?

The best way to answer this question is to give it a shot and study the demographic and personal characteristics of your sample. In one of my online attachment styles questionnaires (http://P034.psch.uic.edu/crq.htm), I found the following demographic breakdowns: The average age of people in my sample is 24 (*SD* = 9), with approximately 80% of the participants being female. An overwhelming proportion are white (70.1%), with Black, Chinese, and Latino being the next three most highly represented ethnic groups. Of my participants who are not from the United States, the majority are from Canada, the United Kingdom, Singapore, and Australia. Finally, approximately 13% of my sample are married. Of those who are not, approximately 59% are in serious relationships.

It should be clear that there is no way to obtain an ideal sample over the Internet (although I'll discuss some possible improvements below). From a practical point of view, one of the critical questions is, How do Internet samples differ from the most common samples used in behavioral science—a student subject pool? Using a student subject pool is fraught with problems, but funding constraints in the behavioral sciences typically leave us with few alternatives.

Internet samples are clearly more restricted than is desirable, because all participants have access to the Internet and are therefore probably more educated than the average person (Reips, 2000). Nonetheless, I believe the Web is probably a better alternative for recruiting participants for many purposes than student subject pools. Respondents are more likely to vary in age, income, country of origin, and occupation. As a result, the data obtained from an Internet sample should be more robust than that obtained from college student samples.

I suspect that many researchers who are reluctant to use the Internet are not resisting it because the Web poses new problems for research, but because it is something new and unfamiliar. Here is an interesting thought experiment. Imagine that you and your colleagues have spent decades recruiting thousands of subjects via the Internet for your research. You're aware of the limitations of recruiting subjects in this manner, but the process is clearly more cost-effective than recruiting a genuinely random sample from the population. Moreover, your sample is composed of people from many walks of life, a wide age range, and different nations. Now, a colleague comes into your office one day and says, "I got a great idea. Instead of recruiting subjects from the Web, let's recruit them from our introductory classes!" You'd probably be flabbergasted by the suggestion, and it is doubtful that you'd be willing to drop your online research to make such a transition.

Of course, part of the resistance isn't due to recruitment or sampling issues per se, but from questions of data quality. When your research subjects are a captive audience from an introductory class in your discipline, you can pretty much ensure that they will complete the experiment—no matter how dull the experiment might be. On the Internet, however, your participants may get bored and drop out midway through your study. I'll discuss some of these concerns below.

Some entrepreneurs have combined the science of sampling with Internet technology. Knowledge Networks (http://www.knowledgenetworks.com/) has drawn a random sample of American families using random digit dialing techniques and has installed free WebTV in their homes. In exchange for free Internet access, the participating families agree to participate in web research once a week. The demographic characteristics of Knowledge Network's panel members closely match those of the U.S. population, as indexed by census data. For a sensible fee, Knowledge Networks will administer your research to its panel, and provide you with the data in a wide array of formats (e.g., Excel, SPSS).

To summarize, recruiting subjects via the WWW should not be viewed as a substitute for the need for good sampling techniques. Nor should it be viewed as appropriate for all research investigations. Some studies (e.g., investigations into descriptive or causal relationships between variables) are clearly better suited for investigation in an Internet sample than others (e.g., investigations into the average income and occupation of Americans). However, given limited resources, it doesn't seem that samples recruited via the WWW would be worse than student subject pools.

DROPOUT

In laboratory experiments, it is unusual for research subjects to withdraw midway through the study. In an online study, however, it is much more likely that people will drop out before the study is complete. Dropout is a problem in all research contexts because, if there are factors that systematically differentiate those who drop out from those who continue, the interpretation of the results is compromised.

Fortunately, you can easily monitor dropout rates during the course of an online experiment. If you create an opening page that saves the user's IP address to a data file, you will be able to separate the number of people who visit your study from the number of people who complete your study. If you're using a multipage study (see Chapter 9), you may be able to use the information you collect early in the study to determine if there are factors that systematically differentiate people who drop from those who do not.

To help minimize dropout, it is wise to keep Internet studies as short as possible. The studies my students and I have run online to date have taken no longer than 10 minutes to complete. Also, as will be discussed below, the better designed your web page, the fewer problems participants have in understanding your research, and the less likely it is that they will drop out. Please see Frick, Bachtiger, and Reips (2001) and Knapp and Heidingsfelder (2001) for an in-depth analysis of dropout.

DATA QUALITY CONTROL

If you have an interesting study or informative website, it is quite likely that the same person may participate more than once. For example, someone might go back and change his or her answers "just to see" how doing so affects the feedback received. Although I believe this kind of exploration on the part of your users is a sign that your website is a good one, you will not want the person's "just to see" data to become part of your data base.

There are a couple of easy ways to handle this problem. First, it is a good idea to include an item somewhere in your in your study that says something like, "I've participated in this research before." You many even want to have the "yes" option to this statement preselected so that respondents have to deliberately deselect it if they have not participated before. Second, if you save the user's IP address along with the his or her data, you can later study the dataset to determine whether you've obtained multiple submissions from the same IP address within the same brief period of time. If you import your data into SPSS, for example, you can easily sort by the IP column and look for repeats of the same address. Keep in mind, however, that not all computers have fixed IP addresses. AOL, for example, often rotates its IP addresses across users, so you don't want to simply flag data from the same IP address unless the data were submitted in rapid succession (i.e., within the same 15 minutes). Another thing to consider is that some computers with fixed addresses are used by more than one person (e.g., computers at libraries, coffee houses, or student computer classrooms). Thus, multiple submissions from the same IP address could conceivably be coming from different people. Despite this possibility, it is probably safer to err on the side of caution and flag multiple submissions from the same IP address within the same window of time.

There may also be cases where you receive more than one submission from the same user because he or she pressed the **Submit** button more than once. Web users forget that once the **Submit** button has been pressed there is often a delay while the server processes their information. If it appears that you're receiving a lot of double-submit cases, you may want to place some text next to your submit button that says something like, "Only press the **Submit** button once. There will probably be a brief delay once you've pressed the button."

There are other ways to help improve the quality of your data. You can determine how long it should take to complete certain trials (see Chapter 13) and flag cases where the user took considerably longer than that. There are some research contexts in which you don't want your subjects going for a cup of coffee in the middle of a trial. In other research, however, the amount of time to complete a trial might not matter too much.

People are fickle when they are surfing the Internet (and maybe otherwise, too). As someone recruiting participants over the Internet, your biggest concern is getting them and keeping them. It is unlikely that people would waste their time in your experiment just to give you bad or silly data. Most people will participate in your study because they are hoping to learn something about themselves. If so, hopefully they will be motivated to respond honestly and accurately.

WEB DESIGN

One of my favorite websites is Web Pages That Suck (http://www.webpagesthatsuck.com) by Vincent Flanders. The objective of his site is to help people learn good web design by studying examples of poor design. If you peruse his site, you'll be surprised by the inane things that web-based retail sites do that can alienate potential customers. As Flanders observes, *anything* (e.g., long download times, confusing navigation, sparse content, annoying pop-up adds) that keeps a visitor from getting what he or she wants from a page provides that visitor with a reason to leave. In the world of online marketing, leaving equals death.

I suspect that the same principle holds true in online research: Anything that gets in the way of your user's ability to participate easily will decrease the likelihood that your user will complete the study. To maximize participation, you should consider the following issues when designing your web studies.

Screen Size

Test the way your website looks in browsers of different screen resolutions. As you may be aware if you're using Windows, you can manually set your virtual screen size by right-clicking on your **Desktop**, choosing the **Properties** option, then selecting **Settings**. About 50% of web users have their monitors set to display their screen at 800 x 600 pixels, although 1024 x 768 is common too (see http://www.thecounter.com/). Personally, I prefer 1280 x 1024 because I like to keep multiple windows open at once. If you design your web pages with a larger screen size than that of your typical user, you might be inadvertently creating a page that is difficult to use. The best solution to this and other possible problems is to play to the lowest common denominator. Test your site with a low screen size (e.g., 800 x 600) and make sure it looks the way you intend.

Figure–Ground Contrast

It is wise to make your text as readable as possible. That probably goes without saying, but there are certain color schemes that look nice (e.g., gray text against white backgrounds) but are not as easy to read. It you want to maximize participation, it is probably best to use black text against a white background.

Don't Use JavaScript

As discussed in the introductory chapter, JavaScript is a programming language that runs on the user's browser. There are a lot of neat things that can be done with JavaScript, including what are called "mouseovers"—commands that cause the browser to display something different when the mouse is moved over a specific part of the page. Unfortunately, due to rivalries between Netscape and Microsoft, different browsers are configured to process JavaScript code differently. Microsoft's Internet Explorer, for example, recognizes some JavaScript codes that Netscape's Navigator will not, and vice versa. Creating a web page that uses scripting compatible with a variety of browsers can be a headache.

Moreover, for better or worse, about 11% of web users have the JavaScript option disabled on their browser (see http://www.thecounter. com/). One reason many users turn the JavaScript option off is that many of the annoying pop-up adds that you see when surfing the Web are generated by these scripts. If it is possible to conduct your research without the use of JavaScript, you should seriously consider doing so.

Test Your Page in Different Browsers

Although the techniques we focused on in this book for presenting information to web users relied on HTML, there can be subtle differences in the way different browsers interpret the same HTML code. It is highly unlikely that this will be a problem for you, but it is always wise to test your research pages in different browsers. In fact, I found one example as I was writing this book of a CGI script whose HTML code was parsed differently by Netscape's Navigator and Microsoft's Explorer. (For the record, Netscape's browser parsed the code incorrectly. Older versions of Netscape do not allow background images to be placed in tables [see Chapter 11].) Again, these kinds of problems should be rare, but it is wise to find them in advance.

Minimize the Need to Click and Scroll

To make it as easy as possible for your subject to participate in your study, you should minimize the need for the subject to scroll. If you're using a questionnaire, for example, make sure the anchors for the scale are clear. Don't force your subject to scroll to the top of a page to remind himself or herself of the appropriate anchors for the scale. You may also want to consider placing only a few questions per page (depending on how lengthy the questions are) and having the subject click on a button to go to the next page. In short, unless your user has a scroll-wheel built into his or her mouse, it will be easier for him or her to click on a button to advance to the next set of questions than to scroll down your page manually. Do whatever seems easiest for your user.

Avoid Jargon

Try to make your Informed Consent as clear as possible. If your IRB permits, try to keep it as simple as you can. The more legalese you add to preliminary pages, the less likely it is that participants will stick around. The goal of your consent form is to explain the objectives of the research as simply and concisely as possible. Anything you do to complicate matters is likely to turn people away.

Avoid Using Plug-Ins

One of the current rages in web design is the use of Macromedia's Flash program. Flash is a remarkable tool for creating animations and interactivity. The program relies on vector-coding, which allows it to animate an image efficiently by stretching and compressing it in a variety of ways. This allows web developers to create graphic intensive web pages that don't consume a lot of memory. I'm a huge fan of Flash, and have experimented with it extensively for research. Unfortunately, standard browsers (i.e., Navigator and Internet Explorer) cannot interpret Flash programs without a special plug-in—a program that interfaces with your browser that needs to be downloaded separately from Macromedia. If your users need the Flash plug-in—or any other plug-in—to use your site, chances are that they will not use your site.

Make Your Site Look Professional

Before I decided to major in psychology, I was a major in media arts. As a result, it is difficult for me to resist the temptation to make avant garde, as opposed to functional and user-friendly, web pages. My inclination is to design the site in a way that seems aesthetically sensible to me, and, if you've ever met a media artist before, you've probably discovered that what is aesthetically pleasing to a media artist is not necessarily pleasing to the rest of the world.

I suspect that, when it comes to scientifically based online research studies, your users are going to want to see a site that looks scholarly and scientific rather than one that looks flashy and fun. I could be wrong, however, and I'm not aware of any research on this issue. Regardless, there is a delicate balance you need to maintain. On the one hand, you want the site to appeal to people's desire to understand themselves. On the other, you don't want your site to be like all the other "pop psychology" sites on the Internet; you want it to be scientific, scholarly, and professional. As a way of striking this balance, in the process of recruiting subjects, you want to appeal to people's need to understand themselves, but also make sure your methods are scientifically defensible. In your debriefing, or feedback, don't make claims that you would-n't make in a scientific journal (e.g., don't infer causation from correlational data).

SUMMARY

I hope you have learned enough to begin creating your own Internet research studies. In this book I was only able to cover some of the basics—just enough to get you up and running. As you continue to explore the use of Perl for conducting online research, you'll discover new and creative ways to collect data online. Please visit the website and the online forum for this book often (http://www.web-research-design.net/). I welcome readers to contribute any scripts they've written that they believe other researchers would find useful, as well as to post questions, suggestions, and tips. Good luck with your CGI scripting!

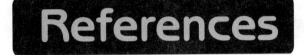

References

Birnbaum, M. H. (2001). *Introduction to behavioral research on the Internet.* Upper Saddle River, NJ: Prentice Hall.

Blascovich, J., & Tomaka, J. (1993). Measures of self-esteem. In J. P. Robinson, P. R. Shaver, & L. S. Wrightsman (Eds.), *Measures of personality and social psychological attitudes* (3rd ed., pp. 115–160). San Diego, CA: Academic Press

Castro, E. (2001). *Perl and CGI for the World Wide Web* (2nd ed.). Berkeley, CA: Peachpit Press.

Epley, N., & Huff, C. W. (1998). Suspicion, affective response, and educational benefit as a result of deception in psychology research. *Personality and Social Psychology Bulletin, 24,* 759–768.

Fraley, R. C., & Shaver, P. R. (2000). Adult romantic attachment: Theoretical developments, emerging controversies, and unanswered questions. *Review of General Psychology, 4,* 132–154.

Frick, A., Bächtiger, M. T., & Reips, U.-D. (2001). Financial incentives, personal information and drop-out in online studies. In U.-D. Reips & M. Bosnjak (Eds.), *Dimensions of Internet science* (pp. 209–219). Lengerich, Germany: Pabst Science Publishers.

Hamilton, J. D. (2000). *CGI programming 101: Perl for the World Wide Web.* Cgi101.com (press).

Knapp, F., & Heidingsfelder, M. (2001). Drop-out analysis: Effects of the survey design. In U.-D. Reips & M. Bosnjak (Eds.), *Dimensions of Internet science* (pp. 221–230). Lengerich, Germany: Pabst Science Publishers.

Reips, U.-D. (2000). The Web experiment method: Advantages, disadvantages, and solutions. In M. H. Birnbaum (Ed.), *Psychological Experiments on the Internet* (pp. 89–117). San Diego, CA: Academic Press.

Rosenberg, M. (1965). *Society and the adolescent self-image*. Princeton, NJ: Princeton University Press.

Shepard, R. N., & Metzler, J. (1971). Mental rotation of three-dimensional objects. *Science, 171,* 701–703.

Index

Symbols

--$i, 198
-, 109
#, 179
$query->end_html, 91, 100, 102
$query->header, 91, 100, 102
$query->param(), 88
$query->redirect(), 149
$query->referer(), 97, 103
$query->remote_addr(), 97, 103
$query->start_html(), 91, 100, 102
$query, 88
 , 43, 58
*, 109
**, 109
**(.5), 109
/, 109
\", 245
\@, 140
\n, 90

+, 109
++$i, 130, 136

HTML Tags

< > </ >, 48–49, 58
<B> </B>, 41, 58
<BODY> </BODY>, 36, 58

, 42, 58
<CENTER> </CENTER>, 43, 58
<FONT> </FONT>, 41–42, 58
<FORM> </FORM>, 60–61, 79
<HTML> </HTML>, 36–37, 58
<I> </I>, 41, 58
<IMG>, 44–48, 58
<INPUT>, 62–71, 79–81
<OPTION> </OPTION>, 67, 80
<P> </P>, 42
<SELECT> </SELECT>, 66–68, 80
<TABLE> </TABLE>, 50–53, 59
<TD> </TD>, 50–51, 59

<TEXTAREA> </TEXTAREA>, 63–64, 79
<TITLE> </TITLE>, 39
<TR> </TR>, 50–51, 59

A

Access log, 276
ActivePerl, 23–24
Addition (*see* Math operators)
Adobe Photoshop, 48
ALIGN, 187
Apache server software, 24
   configuration/running, 26–28, 30, 32
   installing, 24–26
   troubleshooting, 31–32
Append, 89, 166, 173, 223
Array, 132
Averaging scores, 105, 108–110

B

Bar graphs, 182–188
barblack.jpg, 184–185, 187
bargray.jpg, 182–185, 187
Between-subjects manipulations, 146–154
BGCOLOR, 40, 243
Blank space, 43
blank.gif, 190, 192–193
Bold, 41
BORDER, 51
Browser, 4

C

Case sensitive, 272
CELLPADDING, 51–52
CELLSPACING, 51–52

Centering text/images, 43
cgi-bin directory, 20, 30
CGI (common gateway interface), 5, 82
CGI data packet, 88, 99
CGI scripts, 5
CGI.pm, 92, 165, 173
Checkboxes, 68
CHECKED, 66, 80
Client-side programs, 5
close() (Perl), 90, 102
COLOR, 42
Colors in HTML, 40–41
COLSPAN, 52–53
Comma-delimited file, 90, 101
Comment, 179
Conditional branching structures, 174–180

D

Data quality, 282–285
Debriefing, 104–125, 289
Division (*see* Math operators)
dot.gif, 190, 192–193

E

else (Perl), 119
ENCTYPE, 61–62, 71
Environment variables (*see* Variables)
Error log, 276
Ethics, 274–275
example1.htm, 20, 37–38, 49
example2.htm, 39–40, 49
example3.htm, 43
examplesurvey1.htm, 71
Excel, 98–99
Exponent (*see* Math operators)

F

fatalsToBrowser, 269–270
figure1.jpg, 44, 46–47, 57–59
File handle, 89–90
Files, used in programs (*see also* Listings)
   barblack.jpg, 184–185, 187
   bargray.jpg, 182–185, 187
   blank.gif, 190, 192–193
   dot.gif, 190, 192–193
   figure1.jpg, 44, 46–47, 57–59
   image1.jpg, 139–140
   image2.jpg, 139
   image3.jpg, 139
   imagemap1.jpg, 70, 74, 80
   passwords.txt, 205, 207
   relationalstructures.jpg, 49, 54, 75, 83
   scale.jpg, 170
   2dback360.jpg, 190, 192–193
1st Page, 34–36
Flash, 288
flock() (Perl), 90–91, 103
for-next (Perl), 129, 144
foreach (Perl), 114
Formatting text, 41–44
Forms, 60–61, 99
fornextexample1.pl, 129
fornextexample2.pl, 131–132
forumdiscussion.pl, 235–238, 240, 242, 248,
   252, 256–258
forumgototopic.pl, 238, 241, 245–246, 252,
   257
forumnewreply.pl, 249–250, 257–258
forumnewtopic.pl, 235, 242, 246, 254, 257–
   258
forumsavereply.pl, 250–251, 257–258
forumsavetopic.pl, 253–255, 257–258
FTP, 280

G

GD.pm, 181
graph2d.pl, 188–189, 195–196
graph2dsimple.pl, 196
graphbar.pl, 183–184, 187
graphdemo2d.pl, 188, 190, 196
graphdemo2dsimple.pl, 197
graphdemobar.pl, 183, 185

H

HEIGHT, 47
Hexadecimal code, 40–41
Hidden tags, 70–71
   to pass array variables, 165, 173
   to pass scalar variables, 71, 157
home.htm, 55
HTML (hypertext markup language), 4
Hyperlinks, 48–49, 58
   HTML code, 48, 58
   using images as links, 49–50

I

if-else (Perl), 117,118
Image maps, 69–70, 74–75, 80, 167–168,
   171–172
image1.jpg, 139–140
image2.jpg, 139
image3.jpg, 139
imagemap1.jpg, 70, 74, 80
Images, 44–48, 58
   adjusting dimensions, 47–48
   HTML code, 46
   image directory, 44–45
   saving images, 46
Importing data, 98–99
Index variable, 129, 144

index.htm, 55
Informed consent, 274–275, 287
Inserting HTML code, into CGI script, 91–92
Internet Explorer, 4, 6, 7, 286, 287
IP address, 21, 31
  extracting from user, 97
  static, 21
  dynamic, 21
Italics, 41

J

JavaScript, 2, 5–6, 286–287

K

Knowledge Networks, 282–283

L

Line break, 42, 58
Links (*see* Hyperlinks)
Listings (*see also* Files, used in programs)
  example1.htm, 20, 37–38, 49
  example2.htm, 39–40, 49
  example3.htm, 43
  examplesurvey1.htm, 71
  home.htm, 55
  index.htm, 55
  moodsurvey.htm, 74, 77, 83
  moodsurvey2.htm, 73, 86, 92
  randassign-a.htm, 147–149
  randassign-b.htm, 147–149
  self-esteem.htm, 105, 107, 110
  self-esteem2.htm, 111, 114
  self-esteem3.htm, 114, 117–118
  self-esteem4.htm, 118

fornextexample1.pl, 129
fornextexample2.pl, 131–132
forumdiscussion.pl, 235–238, 240, 242, 248, 252, 256–258
forumgototopic.pl, 238, 241, 245–246, 252, 257
forumnewreply.pl, 249–250, 257–258
forumnewtopic.pl, 235, 242, 246, 254, 257–258
forumsavereply.pl, 250–251, 257–258
forumsavetopic.pl, 253–255, 257–258
graph2d.pl, 188–189, 195–196
graph2dsimple.pl, 196
graphbar.pl, 183–184, 187
graphdemo2d.pl, 188, 190, 196
graphdemo2dsimple.pl, 197
graphdemobar.pl, 183, 185
multiform1.pl, 156–160
multiform2.pl, 156–160, 165
onlinequiz.pl, 259–265
pindemo1.pl, 200–203
pindemo2.pl, 203–204, 211–213
pindemosave.pl, 203, 208, 210
pindemosurvey0.pl, 203, 209–210, 213
randassign.pl, 149
randassign2.pl, 151–152
randesteem1.pl, 127, 129, 133, 136–138
randesteem2.pl, 142
randexample.pl, 138
randmultiform1.pl, 163, 166, 171
randmultiform2.pl, 163–165
randmultiform3.pl, 167, 171
randmultiform4.pl, 167–171
rtdemo1.pl, 217, 220–221, 224, 232
rtdemo2.pl, 224, 231–232
rtdemorand1.pl, 226
rtdemorand2.pl, 226–227, 229, 231
savedata1.pl, 83, 86, 93, 98

savedata2.pl, 95–96, 98
self-esteem-coord.pl, 167, 170, 172
self-esteem.pl, 106, 108, 110, 158–159,
    161–162, 165–166
self-esteem2.pl, 111, 114
self-esteem3.pl, 112, 114, 117, 118, 172
self-esteem4.pl, 118, 128, 136–138
skippatterns.pl, 175, 177, 180
Local variable (*see* Variables)
localtime() (Perl), 96
Log files, 276
    access log, 276
    error log, 276
Logical conditions, 120–121
Loop, 114
    for–next (Perl), 129
    foreach (Perl), 114
    while (Perl), 128, 134, 145

M

Macintosh, 4
mailto, 61, 71, 74, 75, 79, 83, 139, 143,
    147–148,152
Math operators, 109
    addition, 109
    division, 109
    exponent, 109
    square root, 109
    subtraction, 109
META tags, 273
METHOD, 61–62, 71
Microsoft's Windows Installer (MSI), 22–23
moodsurvey.htm, 74, 77, 83
moodsurvey2.htm, 73, 86, 92
multiform1.pl, 156–160
multiform2.pl, 156–160, 165
Multiple submissions, 284

Multiplication (*see* Math operators)

N

Nesting, 122, 192, 221
Netfirms, 11
    signing up with Netfirms, 12–13
    transferring files with Netfirms, 13, 15–
    19
Netscape, 6, 193, 286, 287
Non-breaking space, 43, 58

O

onlinequiz.pl, 259–265
open() (Perl), 89–91, 100, 102
Order of operations, 110

P

Paint Shop Pro, 48
password, 81, 204
passwords.txt, 205, 207
Perl, 2, 5, 22–24, 30, 82
Permissions, 279–281
PIN (Personal Identification Number), 3,
    199, 213
pindemo1.pl, 200–203
pindemo2.pl, 203–204, 211–213
pindemosave.pl, 203, 208, 210
pindemosurvey0.pl, 203, 209–210, 213
Plug-ins, 288
post, 61–62
print() (Perl), 90, 102
Public HTML, 19, 55
Publicizing your website, 272
Pull-down menus, 66–68

Q

Quizzes, 14, 258–267
Quotes, 40, 269

R

Radio buttons, 64–66
randassign-a.htm, 147–149
randassign-b.htm, 147–149
randassign.pl, 149
randassign2.pl, 151–152
randesteem1.pl, 127, 129, 133, 136–138
randesteem2.pl, 142
randexample.pl, 138
randmultiform1.pl, 163, 166, 171
randmultiform2.pl, 163–165
randmultiform3.pl, 167, 171
randmultiform4.pl, 167–171
Random assignment, 146–154
    using different pages, 146–150
    within script, 151–153
Randomizing stimuli, 126–145
    examples, 134, 149
    general code, 134
    managing variable names, 135–138
Redirect, 149
Refresh/reload, 38
Registering URL, 272–274
relationalstructures.jpg, 49, 54, 75, 83
Replace carriage return, 254, 277
Response times, 215–232
Reverse key, 109
Rosenberg self-esteem scale, 105
Round, 110
ROWSPAN, 52–53
rtdemo1.pl, 217, 220–221, 224, 232
rtdemo2.pl, 224, 231–232

rtdemorand1.pl, 226
rtdemorand2.pl, 226–227, 229, 231

S

Sampling, 281–283
savedata1.pl, 83, 86, 93, 98
savedata2.pl, 95–96, 98
Saving data, 86–94
    generic, 212, 214
    specific, 89–90
Scalar variable (*see* Variables)
scale.jpg, 170
Screen size, 285–286
Security, 276–281
    personal data security, 278–281
    server security, 276–278
SELECTED, 67, 72, 80
self-esteem-coord.pl, 167, 170, 172
Self-esteem, 105
self-esteem.htm, 105, 107, 110
self-esteem.pl, 106, 108, 110, 158–159,
        161–162, 165–166
self-esteem2.htm, 111, 114
self-esteem2.pl, 111, 114
self-esteem3.htm, 114, 117–118
self-esteem3.pl, 112, 114, 117, 118, 172
self-esteem4.htm, 118
self-esteem4.pl, 118, 128, 136–138
Server-side programs, 5
Server, 4, 24
    creating your own Apache server, 21–32
    setting up, 9–32
    using professional web hosting service,
        11–20
Server maintenance, 275–276
Shebang!, 87
SIZE, 42

Skip patterns, 174–180
skippatterns.pl, 175, 177, 180
Space, 43, 58
split (Perl), 114, 115
sprintf() (Perl), 110
SPSS, 98–99
Square root (*see* Math operators)
srand (Perl), 134
Statelessness, 156
Strings, 120, 135
Submit button, 60–61, 69, 70, 99
Substitution, 110, 124, 135, 140, 183
Subtraction (*see* Math operators)

T

Tables, 50–53, 59
    adjusting cell padding, 51–52
    adjusting cell spacing, 51–52
    adjusting the borders, 51
    creating cells, 50–51, 59
    creating rows, 50–51, 59
    HTML code, 50–51, 59
    spanning rows or columns, 52–53
Text area, 63–64
Text boxes, 62–63
Time, transforming Perl's time format into
    conventional format, 251
Time/timestamping, 95–96
Timing out, 20
Transferring files
    Apache, 28–29, 37–38
    Netfirms, 13, 15–18, 37–38, 92–93

Troubleshooting, 31–32, 94, 268–272
2dback360.jpg, 190, 192–193
Two-dimensional coordinate graphs, 188–
    198

U

Up button, 16
URL (universal resource locator), 4, 19, 29
User, 4

V

Variables, 88–89
    array variable, 89, 103
    environment variable, 88, 97
    local variable, 89
    scalar variable, 89, 102
Virus scans, 21–22

W

Web design, 285–289
What you see is what you get (WYSIWYG),
    33–34
WIDTH, 47
Within-subjects manipulations, 153, 226–
    232
Writing to, text file, 89–91, 100–101
WS_FTP Pro, 13–19, 92–93
WWW (World Wide Web), 5
www directory (*see* Public HTML)